Essentials of ENT Surgical Procedures

Zohaib Siddiqui • Basim Wahba
Keli Dusu
Editors

Essentials of ENT Surgical Procedures

Mastering Key Concepts through Q&A

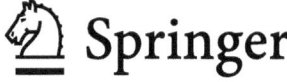

Editors
Zohaib Siddiqui
Medway NHS Foundation Trust
Kent, UK

Basim Wahba
Queen Victoria Hospital
East Grinstead, UK

Keli Dusu
Frimley Park Hospital
Camberley, UK

ISBN 978-3-031-71393-4   ISBN 978-3-031-71394-1   (eBook)
https://doi.org/10.1007/978-3-031-71394-1

© The Editor(s) (if applicable) and The Author(s), under exclusive license to Springer Nature Switzerland AG 2024

This work is subject to copyright. All rights are solely and exclusively licensed by the Publisher, whether the whole or part of the material is concerned, specifically the rights of translation, reprinting, reuse of illustrations, recitation, broadcasting, reproduction on microfilms or in any other physical way, and transmission or information storage and retrieval, electronic adaptation, computer software, or by similar or dissimilar methodology now known or hereafter developed.

The use of general descriptive names, registered names, trademarks, service marks, etc. in this publication does not imply, even in the absence of a specific statement, that such names are exempt from the relevant protective laws and regulations and therefore free for general use.

The publisher, the authors and the editors are safe to assume that the advice and information in this book are believed to be true and accurate at the date of publication. Neither the publisher nor the authors or the editors give a warranty, expressed or implied, with respect to the material contained herein or for any errors or omissions that may have been made. The publisher remains neutral with regard to jurisdictional claims in published maps and institutional affiliations.

This Springer imprint is published by the registered company Springer Nature Switzerland AG
The registered company address is: Gewerbestrasse 11, 6330 Cham, Switzerland

If disposing of this product, please recycle the paper.

Preface

Welcome to this comprehensive guide on otolaryngology (ENT) surgical procedures, designed to serve as a valuable resource for medical professionals at various stages of their careers, from medical students to specialist surgical trainees. This book provides a thorough exploration of key topics within otolaryngology, presenting both foundational knowledge and advanced surgical techniques.

The book covers almost every procedure required to be performed by an ENT specialist, organised into seven distinct chapters: Head and Neck Surgery, Otology, Rhinology, Laryngology, Paediatrics, Emergencies, and Facial Plastics. Each chapter not only describes the procedural steps in detail but also includes potential consultant questions to ensure a thorough understanding of the subject matter. The inclusion of these Q&A sections is intended to foster a deeper knowledge, encourage critical thinking, and prepare practitioners for real-world applications and consultant-level discussions.

This book aims to be an indispensable reference, offering practical insights and up-to-date information to support the ongoing education and development of otolaryngology professionals. Whether you are a student building your foundational skills or an experienced surgeon seeking advanced techniques, this guide is designed to enhance your practice and improve patient care.

Thank you for choosing this book as part of your professional journey.

London, UK	Zohaib Siddiqui
East Grinstead, UK	Basim Wahba
London, UK	Keli Dusu

Acknowledgements

I would like to express my deepest gratitude to the many individuals who have supported me throughout the creation of this book.

First and foremost, I thank God, my wife, and my parents for their unwavering support and encouragement, which has been a constant source of strength and inspiration.

I am profoundly grateful to my teachers and mentors, whose guidance and expertise have been invaluable in shaping my career and this work. I would particularly like to thank Mr. VanWyk, Mr. Hern, Ms. Pitkin, Ms. Molena, Col. Okpala, Ms. Najuko, Mr. Davis, Prof. Kanegaonkar, Mr. Upile, and Mr. Mallick. Your dedication to the field of otolaryngology has been a driving force behind this book.

I would also like to acknowledge my colleagues, peers, and the authors of this book, whose collaboration, feedback, and contributions have enriched this project. Your insights, hard work, and dedication have greatly contributed to the depth and quality of this guide. Additionally, I would like to thank Mr. Vikum Liyanaarachchi for providing the illustrations.

Thank you all for being an integral part of this endeavour.

Contents

1. **Head and Neck** 1
   Ali Al-lami, Zohaib Siddiqui, Basim Wahba, and Keli Dusu

2. **Otology** 51
   Iain Mckay-Davies, Zohaib Siddiqui, Basim Wahba, and Keli Dusu

3. **Rhinology** 91
   Carl van Wyk, Zohaib Siddiqui, Basim Wahba, and Keli Dusu

4. **Laryngology** 127
   Natalie Watson, Zohaib Siddiqui, Basim Wahba, and Keli Dusu

5. **Paediatrics** 145
   Kiran Varadharajan, Zohaib Siddiqui, Basim Wahba, and Keli Dusu

6. **Emergencies** 165
   Sameer Mallick, Zohaib Siddiqui, Basim Wahba, and Keli Dusu

7. **Facial Plastics** 219
   Sami AlHassan, Zohaib Siddiqui, Basim Wahba, and Keli Dusu

Editors and Contributors

Editors

Zohaib Siddiqui Medway NHS Foundation Trust, Kent, UK

Basim Wahba Queen Victoria Hospital, East Grinstead, UK
Faculty of Medicine, Cairo University, Giza, Egypt

Keli Dusu Frimley Park Hospital, Camberley, UK

Contributors

Sami AlHassan The Royal London Hospital, London, UK

Ali Al-lami East Kent Hospitals University, Kent and Canterbury Hospital, Canterbury, Kent, UK

Keli Dusu Frimley Park Hospital, Camberley, UK

Sameer Mallick Nottingham University Hospital, Nottingham, UK

Iain Mckay-Davies Maidstone and Tunbridge Wells Hospital, Maidstone, UK

Zohaib Siddiqui Medway NHS Foundation Trust, Kent, UK

Kiran Varadharajan Royal Surrey County Hospital, Guildford, UK

Basim Wahba Queen Victoria Hospital, East Grinstead, UK
Faculty of Medicine, Cairo University, Giza, Egypt

Natalie Watson Guy's and St Thomas NHS Foundation Trust, St Thomas' Hospital, London, UK

Carl van Wyk Frimley Park Hospital, Frimley, Camberley, UK

Illustrators

Vikum Liyanaarachchi University of Colombo, Colombo, Sri Lanka

Zohaib Siddiqui Medway NHS Foundation Trust, Kent, UK

Head and Neck

Ali Al-lami, Zohaib Siddiqui, Basim Wahba, and Keli Dusu

1.1 Thyroidectomy

Indications for Surgery [1]
Indications for thyroid surgery can be remembered as the 4 Cs: cancer, control of thyrotoxicosis, compression, and cosmesis.

- Benign thyroid nodules causing compressive symptoms or cosmetic concerns
- Thyrotoxicosis including Graves' diseases, toxic multinodular goitre, or toxic adenoma causing hyperthyroidism
- Thyroid cancer (papillary, follicular, medullary, or anaplastic)
- Retrosternal goitre causing tracheal compression
- Suspected malignancy based on fine needle aspiration biopsy (FNAB) or indeterminate cytology

Specific Risks Involved with the Surgery
Can be divided into immediate, early, and late.
  Immediate

A. Al-lami (✉)
East Kent Hospitals University, Kent and Canterbury Hospital, Canterbury, Kent, UK
e-mail: ali.al-lami@nhs.net

Z. Siddiqui
Medway NHS Foundation Trust, Gillingham, Kent, UK

B. Wahba
Queen Victoria Hospital, East Grinstead, West Sussex, UK

K. Dusu
Frimley Park Hospital, Frimley, Camberley, UK

© The Author(s), under exclusive license to Springer Nature Switzerland AG 2024
Z. Siddiqui et al. (eds.), *Essentials of ENT Surgical Procedures*, https://doi.org/10.1007/978-3-031-71394-1_1

- Recurrent laryngeal nerve (RLN) injury: temporary, permanent
- Hypoparathyroidism (leading to hypocalcemia): temporary, permanent
- Hypothyroidism (if hemithyroidectomy, 20% chance)
- Hematoma: may require urgent surgical intervention
- Superior laryngeal nerve injury
- Tracheomalacia

Early (days–weeks)

- Infection
- Aspiration secondary to vocal cord palsy

Late

- Scarring and keloid formation

Steps of the Surgery

1. Administer general anaesthesia and endotracheal intubation.
2. Position the patient supine with a rolled towel or shoulder roll to extend the neck. Use a head ring to support the head.
3. Place the leads required for the RLN monitor. Prep + drape the patient.
4. Consider injecting local anaesthetic such as Lignospan (1:80,000 adrenaline) or 1:100,000 adrenaline for haemostasis.
5. Perform a transverse curvilinear skin incision midway between the cricoid cartilage and the sternal notch, curving slightly upward (ideally using an existing skin crease).
6. Dissect subplatysmal flaps superiorly and inferiorly to expose the strap muscles. Use cold-steel or mono-polar dissection. Use the anterior jugular veins as your deep margin. Superiorly, you would raise the flap until you are able to palpate the thyroid cartilage. Inferiorly, it should be until the clavicle.
7. Use instruments such as fishhooks, sutures, Alexis retractor, or a Joll's retractor to expose the surgical field.
8. If a continuous intraoperative nerve monitor for the RLN is used, at this point, you would dissect and present the vagus nerve (found in the carotid sheath between and posterior to the common carotid artery and internal jugular vein) and clip the monitor to the nerve.
9. Divide through the midline down to thyroid isthmus, and retract the strap muscles to expose the thyroid gland, as seen in Fig. 1.1. If required, transect the sterno-thyroid or sterno-hyoid strap muscles for superior access for the superior pole of the thyroid gland.
10. Start by dissecting out the superior pole of the thyroid gland. Stick close to the thyroid gland capsule, and dissect the vasculature as required. Dissecting Joll's triangle between thyroid and trachea can be useful.

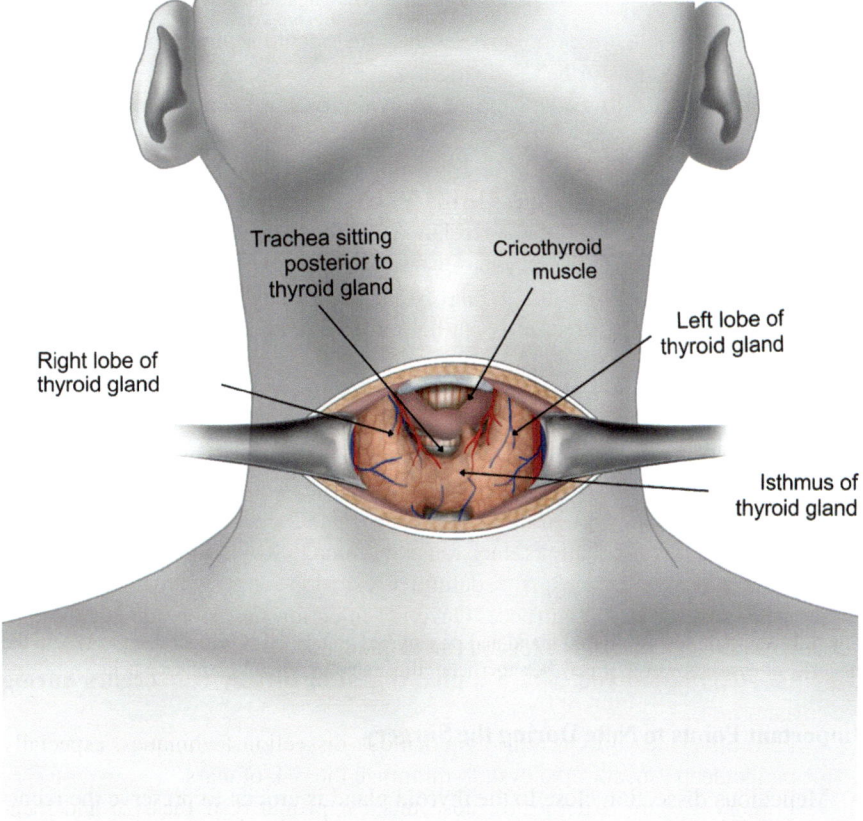

Fig. 1.1 Thyroid anatomy. Illustrated by Vikum Liyanaarachchi

11. Identify and preserve the superior parathyroid glands and their blood supply with meticulous dissection (Fig. 1.2).
12. Continue the dissection by focussing on the inferior pole. Carefully dissect to preserve the blood supply of the parathyroid glands.
13. Identify and ligate the superior, middle thyroid vein and inferior thyroid vessels.
14. Identify and preserve the recurrent laryngeal nerve, and confirm its position using the nerve monitor. This requires careful dissection in the tracheo-oesophageal groove at the level of the cricothyroid joint.
15. If total thyroidectomy, repeat this procedure on the opposite side and remove the thyroid gland (either a hemithyroidectomy or total thyroidectomy, depending on the indication).
16. Achieve meticulous haemostasis with a head down and Valsalva, and inspect the surgical field. You may place haemostatic soluble material in the surgical site, and cover the RLN.
17. If required, insert suction drain (i.e. large dead space or a prior oozing operation).
18. Close the strap muscles, platysma, and skin in layers using appropriate sutures.

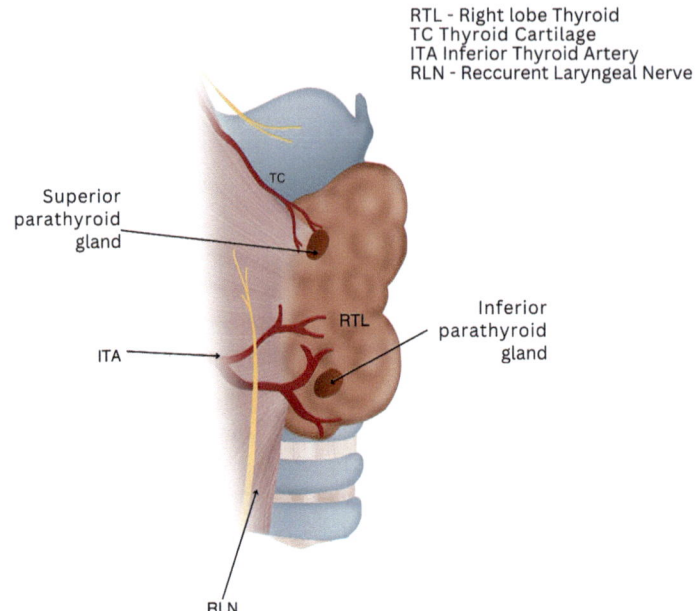

Fig. 1.2 Sagittal view of thyroid gland and parathyroid glands. RLN will sit deep to ITA in the majority of cases; however, it may be superficial. Illustrated by Vikum Liyanaarachchi

Important Points to Note During the Surgery

- Meticulous dissection close to the thyroid gland is crucial to preserve the recurrent laryngeal nerve and parathyroid glands and its blood supply; Fig. 1.3 shows the arterial supply to this region.
- Use intraoperative nerve monitoring if available to help identify and protect the recurrent laryngeal nerve. Consider continuous nerve monitoring.
- Inspect the surgical field carefully for haemostasis to prevent post-operative haematoma.
- If performing a total thyroidectomy for cancer, consider central compartment lymph node dissection based on the extent of the disease.

Questions a Consultant Might Ask a Trainee About the Operation

1. **What are the surgical landmarks of the recurrent laryngeal nerve?**

    The recurrent laryngeal nerve (RLN) is located in the tracheo-oesophageal groove and inserts into the cricothyroid joint [2]. In 50% of patients, it is found deep to the inferior thyroid artery (ITA); in 25%, it is between the ITA branches, and in another 25%, it lies anterior to the ITA. The RLN is also in close proximity to the tubercle of Zuckerkandl, typically posteromedial. Posterior to the cricothyroid joint, the nerve inserts into the larynx. The right RLN has a more

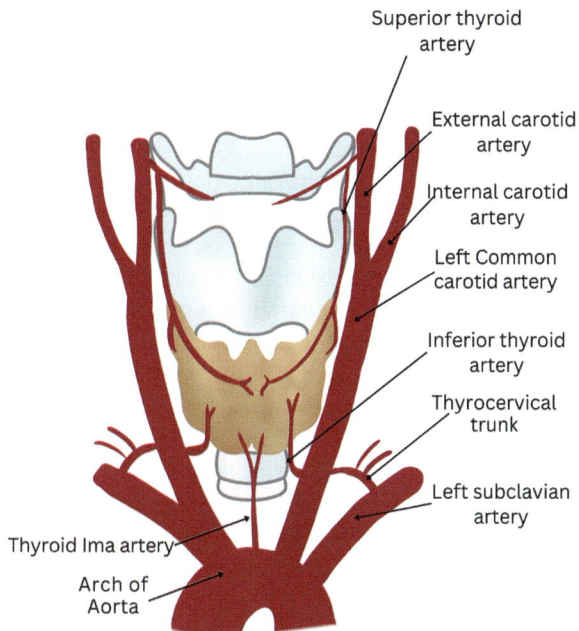

Fig. 1.3 Arterial blood supply to thyroid gland. Illustrated by Vikum Liyanaarachchi

oblique path compared to the left, as it loops around the right subclavian artery, while the left RLN loops around the aortic arch.

2. **When do you expect a non-recurrent laryngeal nerve?**

    A non-recurrent laryngeal nerve is rare, occurring in <1% of cases, and almost always on the right side [2]. You might expect it before surgery if an X-ray or CT scan shows an aberrant subclavian artery (arteria lusoria), where the right subclavian artery arises from the aortic arch. In such cases, the laryngeal nerve does not loop around the subclavian artery but instead arises directly from the vagus nerve in a non-recurrent fashion.

3. **What are Joll's triangle and Beahrs' triangle?**

    Joll's triangle is used to identify the external branch of the superior laryngeal nerve (SLN). It is bounded medially by the midline (trachea), laterally by the superior pole of the thyroid, and superiorly by the strap muscles' attachment. Beahrs' triangle helps identify the recurrent laryngeal nerve (RLN). The common carotid artery (CCA) forms the base, the inferior thyroid artery (ITA) forms one side, and the RLN itself forms the other side of the triangle.

4. **How do you manage a haematoma post-thyroidectomy?**

    Management can be either conservative or surgical, depending on the rate of haematoma expansion and whether there is airway compromise. If intervention is needed, the SCOOP protocol should be performed: remove Steri-Strips, cut sutures, open the skin, open the muscles, and pack the wound. The consultant and anaesthetists should be informed, and a flexible nasal endoscopy (FNE) should be done to assess the difficulty of intubation, as laryngeal oedema is often expected in these cases.

5. **How do you manage a thyrotoxic storm?**

   Managing a thyrotoxic storm is an emergency procedure often necessary in cases of uncontrolled thyrotoxicosis, where a surge of thyroxine hormones enters the bloodstream. This requires a multidisciplinary team approach, involving senior anaesthetic, endocrinology, intensive care unit (ICU), and ENT specialists. Symptoms to expect include tachycardia, arrhythmias, hyperthermia, hypertension, confusion, and potentially coma. Treatment includes administering IV fluids, IV steroids, cooling measures, IV propranolol, potassium iodide (KI), or sodium iodide (NaI) and admitting the patient to the ICU.

6. **What are the landmarks for your incision, and why did you choose this specific location?**

   The landmarks for the incision include the sternal notch and the cricoid cartilage. The incision is typically made midpoint between the cricoid cartilage and the sternal notch, about two fingerbreadths above the sternal notch, curving slightly upward [1]. This location is chosen because it provides optimal exposure of the thyroid gland while minimizing the visible scar. Aligning with the natural skin creases further reduces the scar's appearance post-operatively.

7. **How can you differentiate the parathyroid glands from the surrounding tissue, and why is it essential to preserve them?**

   The parathyroid glands are small, yellowish-brown, ovoid structures usually located on the posterior aspect of the thyroid gland. They can be distinguished from surrounding fatty and lymphatic tissues by their distinct colour and shape [3]. Preserving the parathyroid glands is crucial because they regulate calcium homeostasis. Damage to their blood supply or removal can cause hypoparathyroidism, leading to hypocalcaemia, which may result in serious complications such as tetany, seizures, and cardiac arrhythmias.

8. **Describe the anatomical course of the recurrent laryngeal nerve and its relationship to the thyroid gland.**

   The recurrent laryngeal nerve (RLN) branches from the vagus nerve on each side of the neck. On the right side, it loops around the right subclavian artery and ascends towards the larynx; on the left, it loops around the aortic arch [2]. The RLN then travels between the trachea and oesophagus, running in the tracheo-oesophageal groove. Near the larynx, it courses close to the posterior aspect of the thyroid gland, often passing through Berry's ligament or posterior to the cricothyroid joint (through the fibres of the inferior constrictor muscle). The RLN innervates all intrinsic muscles of the larynx, except the cricothyroid muscle. Preserving the RLN during thyroidectomy is essential to prevent vocal cord paralysis and subsequent hoarseness, dysphonia, or aspiration.

9. **What measures can you take to minimize the risk of post-operativehaematoma?**

   To minimize the risk of post-operative haematoma, meticulous haemostasis is crucial during surgery, ensuring careful ligation or cauterization of blood vessels. Thoroughly inspect the surgical field for any bleeding points before closing, preferably with the patient in a head-down position and performing a Valsalva manoeuvre to increase pressure and visualize bleeding points. Place absorbable haemostatic material to aid in clotting. Consider placing a temporary drain to remove any accumulated blood or fluid, and use appropriate suturing techniques to securely close the surgical site. Post-operatively, instruct the patient to avoid activities that could increase blood pressure or strain the neck area.

10. **In cases of thyroid cancer, when would you consider performing a central compartment lymph node dissection?**

    A central compartment lymph node dissection, or central neck dissection, may be considered in thyroid cancer cases when there is evidence of clinically positive lymph nodes in the central compartment (levels VI and VII) on preoperative imaging or physical examination. Other considerations include a primary tumour that is high risk or has aggressive features such as extrathyroidal extension, vascular invasion, or positive margins. Additionally, a history of radiation exposure, a strong family history of thyroid cancer, a primary tumour larger than 4 cm, or bilateral multifocal disease may also warrant this procedure. It is essential to weigh the potential benefits of central compartment lymph node dissection against the risk of complications, such as injury to the recurrent laryngeal nerve and parathyroid glands.

1.2 Parathyroidectomy

Indications for Surgery [4]

- Primary hyperparathyroidism with symptomatic hypercalcaemia.
- Secondary parathyroid hyperplasia in patients with chronic kidney disease.
- Asymptomatic primary hyperparathyroidism with indications for surgery (e.g. serum calcium >1 mg/dL above the upper limit of normal, reduced creatinine clearance, osteoporosis, or nephrolithiasis).
- Recurrent or persistent hyperparathyroidism after previous parathyroid surgery.
- Parathyroid carcinoma or atypical adenoma.
- Tertiary hyperparathyroidism.

Specific Risks Involved with the Surgery
Immediate

- Recurrent laryngeal nerve injury: temporary, permanent
- Hypoparathyroidism: temporary, permanent
- Haematoma: may require urgent surgical intervention
- Failure to identify the site of parathyroid adenoma

Early (days–weeks)

- Hungry bone syndrome
- Infection

Late (months+)

- Scarring and keloid formation
- Persistent or recurrent hyperparathyroidism

Steps of the Surgery (Central Neck Approach)

1. Administer general anaesthesia and monitored endotracheal intubation if RLN monitor is used.
2. Position the patient supine with a rolled towel or shoulder roll and head ring to extend the neck.
3. Place the leads required for the RLN monitor. Prep + drape the patient.
4. Consider Injecting local anaesthetic such as Lignospan (1:80,000 adrenaline) or 1:100,000 adrenaline for haemostasis.
5. Perform a transverse curvilinear skin incision at the midpoint between the cricoid cartilage and sternal notch or 2 fingerbreadths above the sternal notch, curving slightly upward (ideally using an existing skin crease).
6. Dissect subplatysmal flaps superiorly and inferiorly to expose the strap muscles. Use cold-steel or mono-polar dissection.
7. Use instruments such as fishhooks, sutures, Alexis, or a Joll's retractor to expose the surgical field.
8. Divide through the midline down to thyroid isthmus, and retract the strap muscles to expose the thyroid gland. If required, transect the sterno-thyroid or sterno-hyoid strap muscles for superior access for the superior pole of the thyroid gland.
9. If parathyroid adenoma is localized in preoperative imaging, target the relevant quadrant of the parathyroid adenoma.
10. Consider exploring the other ipsilateral parathyroid gland if adenoma is not localized.
11. Identify the parathyroid glands (usually four) and the abnormal gland(s) based on preoperative localization studies or intraoperative findings.
12. If parathyroid adenoma is not easily localized, consider hiding places for an adenoma in the carotid sheath or retro-oesophageal region.
13. Excise the abnormal parathyroid gland(s) while preserving the normal glands and their blood supply.
14. Identify and preserve the recurrent laryngeal nerve.
15. If possible, confirm the excised gland's identity by sending a sample for frozen section or assessing a drop in intraoperative parathyroid hormone (PTH) levels.
16. Achieve meticulous haemostasis, and inspect the surgical field.
17. Consider inserting suction drain if large dead space operating field.
18. Close the strap muscles, platysma, and skin in layers using appropriate sutures.

Important Points to Note During the Surgery

- Meticulous dissection is crucial to identify and preserve the normal parathyroid glands and their blood supply, which includes the inferior and superior thyroid arteries (Figs. 1.2 and 1.3).
- Use intraoperative nerve monitoring if available to help identify and protect the recurrent laryngeal nerve.
- Consider using intraoperative PTH monitoring to confirm successful removal of the abnormal gland(s) and predict post-operative calcium levels.
- Inspect the surgical field carefully for haemostasis to prevent post-operative haematoma.

Questions a Consultant Might Ask a Trainee About the Operation

1. **What are the indications for parathyroidectomy in patients with primary hyperparathyroidism?**
   Parathyroidectomy is indicated in patients with primary hyperparathyroidism for the following reasons: a. Symptomatic hypercalcemia: Patients experiencing symptoms such as fatigue, weakness, depression, bone pain, or kidney stones due to high calcium levels. b. Asymptomatic hyperparathyroidism with indications for surgery: Patients without symptoms but with findings indicating a need for intervention. These may include serum calcium levels >1 mg/dL above the upper limit of normal, reduced creatinine clearance, osteoporosis (T-score ≤ -2.5), nephrolithiasis (kidney stones), or a history of fragility fractures. c. Recurrent or persistent hyperparathyroidism after previous parathyroid surgery: Patients who continue to have elevated parathyroid hormone (PTH) and calcium levels after an initial parathyroidectomy, or those who experience a recurrence. d. Parathyroid carcinoma or atypical adenoma: Patients with malignant or atypical parathyroid tumours [4].

2. **What is the workup before proceeding with parathyroid surgery for primary hyperparathyroidism?**
   This should be done in a multidisciplinary team (MDT) fashion with endocrinology input beforehand:
   As per NICE guidelines 2019 [5]:
   PTH, albumin-adjusted calcium, Vit D, eGFR and creatinine, 24-h urinary calcium, DEXA scan, renal U/S scan, U/S scan neck, and consider sestamibi scan. 4D CT is also being used where available to help localize the adenoma.

3. **What is the reason for requesting 24-h urinary calcium in this setting?**
   To rule out familial hypocalciuric hypercalcaemia. This genetic condition is characterized by high levels of calcium in the blood but low levels of calcium in the urine. Differentiating FHH from primary hyperparathyroidism is crucial, as FHH generally requires conservative management, whereas primary hyperparathyroidism often necessitates surgical intervention.

4. **What is the management if hypocalcaemia develops post-operatively?**
   This should be managed in an MDT approach with endocrinology input:

As per BAETS guidelines [6]:
- If Ca < = 1.8 or severe symptoms: IV calcium gluconate 10% 10 mL in 100 mL saline over 1 h.
- If Ca 1.8–2: calcium tablets (recheck Ca every 12 h) and check/correct Mg.
- If Ca 2–2.1 with symptoms: calcium tablets (recheck Ca every 12 h) and check/correct Mg.
- If Ca 2–2.1 asymptomatic: recheck Ca after 24 h.

5. **What is the embryological origin of parathyroid glands?**

    Superior parathyroid gland originates from the fourth branchial pouch. Inferior parathyroid gland originates from the third branchial pouch [4].

6. **What are the ectopic sites for parathyroid gland (hidden sites)?**

    Superior parathyroid ectopic sites: tracheoesophageal groove, retro-oesophageal, or posterior mediastinum.

    Inferior parathyroid ectopic sites: within thymus, the anterior mediastinum, intrathyroidal, or within thyro-thymic ligament.

    The inferior parathyroid adenoma generally shows a more variable location as it has a longer space to descend into the neck arising from the third branchial arch.

7. **How do you differentiate normal from abnormal parathyroid glands during surgery?**

    Normal parathyroid glands are typically small, yellowish-brown, and ovoid, measuring about 3–4 mm in thickness and 6 mm in length [4]. Abnormal parathyroid glands, such as those affected by adenomas or hyperplasia, are generally larger, with a different texture and colour compared to normal glands. Preoperative localization studies (e.g. sestamibi scan, ultrasound, or 4D CT) and intraoperative findings can help identify the abnormal gland(s). In some cases, intraoperative PTH monitoring can be utilized to confirm successful removal of the abnormal gland(s) and predict post-operative calcium levels.

8. **Describe the anatomical relationship between the parathyroid glands, the thyroid gland, and the recurrent laryngeal nerve.**

    The parathyroid glands are typically located on the posterior aspect of the thyroid gland. There are usually four glands, with two superior and two inferior glands on each side. However, their exact location may vary. The recurrent laryngeal nerve (RLN) runs near the thyroid gland, coursing between the trachea and oesophagus in the tracheoesophageal groove [4]. As it approaches the larynx, the RLN often penetrates the Berry's ligament on the posterior aspect of the thyroid gland. It is essential to preserve the RLN during surgery to prevent vocal cord paralysis and other complications.

    Superior parathyroid glands are typically antero-medial to the RLN. Inferior parathyroid glands are typically postero-lateral to the RLN.

9. **What are the potential complications of parathyroidectomy, and how can you minimize their occurrence?**

    Potential complications of parathyroidectomy include recurrent laryngeal nerve injury, hypoparathyroidism, haematoma, infection, scarring, hungry bone syndrome, and persistent or recurrent hyperparathyroidism. To minimize these complications, a. use meticulous dissection techniques to identify and preserve the normal parathyroid glands, their blood supply, and the recurrent laryngeal nerve; b. utilize intraoperative nerve monitoring, if available, to help identify and protect the recurrent laryngeal nerve; c. achieve thorough haemostasis during surgery, and inspect the surgical field carefully before closing to prevent post-operative haematoma; d. maintain aseptic technique throughout the procedure to minimize the risk of infection; and e. consider using intraoperative PTH monitoring to confirm successful removal of the abnormal gland(s) and predict post-operative calcium levels.

10. **How can intraoperative PTH monitoring be utilized during parathyroidectomy, and what are its benefits?**

    Intraoperative PTH monitoring involves measuring the patient's parathyroid hormone (PTH) levels during the surgery. A baseline PTH level is obtained before the removal of the abnormal parathyroid gland. After excision of the suspected abnormal gland(s), additional PTH samples are taken at specific time intervals, usually 5 and 10 min post-excision. A significant drop in PTH levels (typically more than 50% from the baseline) indicates the successful removal of the hyperfunctioning gland(s).

    The benefits of intraoperative PTH monitoring include (a) confirmation of successful removal of the abnormal parathyroid gland(s) during surgery, reducing the risk of persistent hyperparathyroidism; (b) identification of additional hyperfunctioning glands not detected preoperatively or during the surgery, improving the likelihood of a successful operation; (c) reducing the need for extensive neck exploration, which can minimize the risk of complications such as injury to the recurrent laryngeal nerve and parathyroid glands; (d) providing guidance on the appropriate extent of surgery in cases of multiglandular disease, helping to avoid over- or under-treatment; and (e) allowing for a more accurate prediction of post-operative calcium levels, which can help guide post-operative calcium supplementation and monitoring.

1.3   Neck Dissection (Selective, Modified Radical, Radical)

Indications for Surgery [7]

- Therapeutic: Metastatic cervical lymph node involvement in head and neck malignancies (required to stage the patient's TNM)
- Therapeutic: Nodal recurrence after previous treatment (surgery, radiation, or chemoradiation)
- Elective: Prophylactic treatment for patients with a high risk of occult cervical metastasis
- Salvage surgery for residual or recurrent disease after chemoradiation
- For access purposes when neck vessels need to prepare for microvascular free flap reconstruction

Specific Risks Involved with the Surgery

- Neural injury:
  - Spinal accessory nerve: inability to raise arm/shrug
  - Hypoglossal: tongue weakness
  - Marginal mandibular nerve: lower lip droop
  - Vagus: voice change/swallowing difficulties/altered heart rate
  - Great auricular nerve: numb earlobe
  - Cervical plexus: numbness around neck
  - Phrenic nerve: respiratory difficulties due to reduced diaphragm movement
  - Brachial plexus: weakness of arm movements
  - Horner's syndrome from sympathetic chain injury (ptosis, miosis + anhidrosis)
- Chyle leak
- Haematoma
- Infection
- Seroma
- Skin flap necrosis
- Facial or neck oedema and fibrosis
- Scar/keloid
- Injury of vascular structures: internal jugular vein (IJV) or carotid

Steps of the Surgery (Selective, Modified Radical, Radical Neck Dissection)

1. Administer general anaesthesia and endotracheal intubation.
2. Position the patient supine, with the head turned away from the side to be dissected, and extend the neck with a shoulder roll.
3. Consider nerve monitoring.
4. Multiple incisions are available including utility, hockey-stick, or J-shaped incision. Make a skin incision along the anterior border of the sternocleidomastoid muscle (SCM), starting from the mastoid tip and extending down to the midline of the neck (J incision if one sided; apron incision if bilateral).
5. Consider injecting local anaesthetic such as Lignospan (1:80,000 adrenaline) or 1: 100,000 pure adrenaline for haemostasis.
6. Develop subplatysmal skin flaps superiorly and inferiorly to expose the underlying platysma muscle and the neck's superficial layer.
7. Perform selective, modified radical, or radical neck dissection based on the preoperative assessment and intraoperative findings (Fig. 1.4):
   (a) Selective neck dissection: Remove specific lymph node levels or groups based on the primary tumour's location and risk of metastasis, preserving non-lymphatic structures (e.g. SCM, internal jugular vein, spinal accessory nerve). A level 2-4 dissection begins by skeletonizing the anterior SCM to expose and trace the accessory nerve, noting its proximity to the IJV. Use the digastric's posterior belly as a landmark for the upper limit of level 2a. Clear level 2b within boundaries and proceed to level 2a, keeping tissue intact for an en-bloc

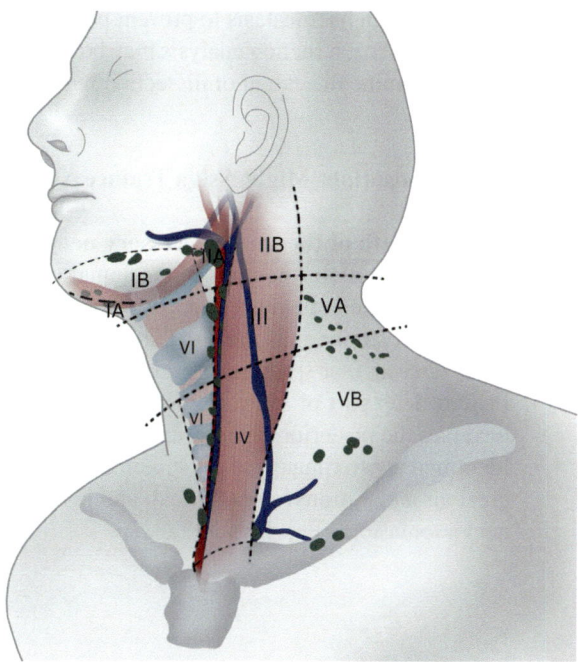

Fig. 1.4 Anatomical levels of the neck (Ia, Ib, IIa, IIb, III, IV, Va, Vb, VI). Illustrated by Vikum Liyanaarachchi

specimen. Free attachments along the SCM and dissect the neck floor, lifting tissue en-bloc. Rotate the specimen over the IJV, skeletonizing it fully without separating lymphatic groups. In level 4, follow the IJV from the clavicle, avoiding the thoracic duct on the left to prevent chyle leaks. Preserve the phrenic nerve on scalenus anterior, carotid artery, vagus nerve, and brachial plexus. Complete levels 2-4 with intact tissue for pathology.
 (b) Modified radical neck dissection: Remove all lymph nodes in the neck's lateral compartment (levels I–V), preserving one structure (type I), two structures (type II), three structures (type III/functional), or more non-lymphatic structures.
 (c) Radical neck dissection: Remove all lymph nodes in the neck's lateral compartment (levels I–V) along with the SCM, internal jugular vein, and spinal accessory nerve.
8. Ensure meticulous haemostasis, and inspect the surgical field.
9. Close the wound in layers using appropriate sutures, and place a drain if necessary.

Important Points to Note During the Surgery

- Careful dissection and identification of critical structures, such as the spinal accessory nerve, internal jugular vein, and carotid artery, are essential to minimize complications (Fig. 1.5).
- Preserve the non-lymphatic structures whenever possible, depending on the extent of the disease and the type of neck dissection performed.

- Achieve thorough haemostasis to prevent post-operative haematoma.
- Intraoperative frozen section analysis may be used to assess the margins of resection and determine the extent of dissection required.

Questions a Consultant Might Ask a Trainee About the Operation

1. **What is the path of the spinal accessory nerve?**
   - Derived from motor neurons in the spinal nucleus down to C5 level. Enters through foramen magnum, and exits via jugular foramen [8]
   - May exit posterior and lateral to the internal jugular vein (commonly), medial (30% of cases), or splitting the vein (3–5% of cases)
   - Pierces deep part of sternocleidomastoid around C2 level, exits posteriorly, traverses the posterior triangle, and innervates the trapezius muscle
   - Identified approximately 1 cm superior to the emergence (Erb's) point of the great auricular, transverse cervical, and lesser occipital nerves from the sternocleidomastoid (Fig. 1.5)

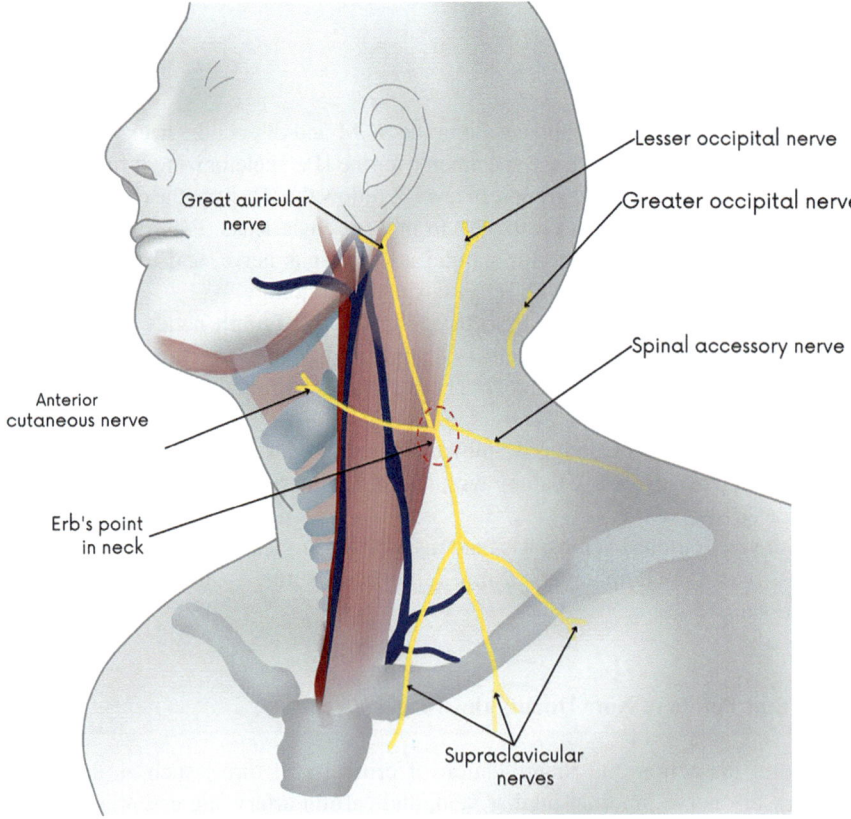

Fig. 1.5 Erb's point demonstrated in the neck. Illustrated by Vikum Liyanaarachchi

2. **How will you manage a chyle leakage intraoperatively?**
   - To manage an intraoperative chyle leak, position the patient's head down and perform the Valsalva maneuver to locate the leak. Use loupe magnification for precise identification, avoid diathermy, and instead ligate or oversew the ducts with tissue glue if needed. Postoperatively, apply a compression dressing, elevate the head, consult a dietitian for a low-fat diet or TPN, consider octreotide to reduce lymph flow, and monitor the drain for milky fluid. For large leaks, check for chylothorax with a chest X-ray.
3. **How would you manage a patient who suffers from a carotidblowout?**
   If palliative setting: Good communication with the patient and family is key. Both should be aware of the possibility and what that might entail. Supportive palliative care should include sedation and pain relief if a blowout occurs. Ideally, follow the local guidelines in terms of medications given to the patient, to allow for a less traumatic ending to life.

   If curative setting: Inform the patient and nursing staff of what may occur. Observe any impending signs, e.g. early signs of bleeding or a herald bleed. An ABCDE approach is important, and preparation is key. Airway: The patient should have a cuffed tracheostomy, to be inflated if bleeding occurs to protect the airway. Bleeding: Immediate compression and packing should be performed. Circulation: Use large-bore canula, fluids/blood, and cross match/G&S (already prepared). Patient should be taken to theatre for surgical ligation or early liaison with vascular team/IR team to assist with possible ablation.
4. **What is the boundary between levels Va and Vb?**
   According to the AJCC classification [9], the two levels are separated by the horizontal plane marking the inferior border of the cricoid cartilage. Va includes the spinal accessory nerve.
5. **What incisions would you prefer in patients who have undergone radiotherapy?**
   There are different named incisions. Though modified Schobinger's and apron incisions are commonly used in neck dissection due to good exposure, they are not the preferred incisions in such cases as the trifurcation point of incision is lying close to carotid sheath. Lahey's lateral utility incision is preferable as it is a posteriorly based incision which avoids a trifurcation point over carotid. Other incisions, e.g. MacFee incisions (double incision), are not commonly used as they give limited exposure, though no intersection points. There are other different incisions, e.g. Conley or H-incision.
6. **Can you describe the differences between selective, modified radical, and radical neck dissections?**
   Selective neck dissection removes specific lymph node levels or groups based on the primary tumour's location and risk of metastasis, preserving non-lymphatic structures. Modified radical neck dissection removes all lymph nodes in the neck's lateral compartment (levels I–V) while preserving one or more non-lymphatic structures. Radical neck dissection removes all lymph nodes in the lateral compartment along with the SCM, internal jugular vein, and spinal accessory nerve [7].

7. **What are the key anatomical landmarks and structures to identify and preserve during a neck dissection, and how can you minimize the risk of injuring these structures?**

   Key anatomical landmarks and structures to identify and preserve during a neck dissection include the spinal accessory nerve, internal jugular vein, and carotid artery. To minimize the risk of injury, use meticulous dissection techniques, provide adequate exposure of the surgical field, and ensure proper identification and handling of these structures. Knowledge of the levels and boundaries of the neck is key (Table 1.1).

8. **What is the importance of post-operative neck imaging and adjuvant therapy in the management of patients undergoing neck dissection for head and neck malignancies?**

   Post-operative neck imaging, such as CT or MRI and PET/CT, can help assess the completeness of the neck dissection, detect residual or recurrent disease, and guide the need for further intervention or adjuvant therapy. Adjuvant therapy, including radiation therapy, chemotherapy, or targeted therapy, may be indicated

Table 1.1 Anatomical levels of the neck and their boundaries with key structures [7]

Level	Name	Boundaries (anatomical)	Subdivisions and notes	Key structures
Ia	Submental triangle	Anterior belly of the digastric muscle, hyoid bone		Lymph nodes, small veins
Ib	Submandibular triangle	Body of the mandible, anterior and posterior bellies of the digastric muscle		Submandibular gland, facial artery and vein, lingual nerve, hypoglossal nerve
II	Upper jugular nodes	Anterior: Stylohyoid muscle border, posterior: Sternocleidomastoid muscle's posterior border. Superior: Skull base. Inferior: Hyoid bone (clinical), carotid bifurcation (surgical)	Divided by the accessory nerve into IIa (anteriorly) and IIB (posteriorly)	Accessory nerve, internal jugular vein, carotid arteries, cranial nerve XI
III	Middle jugular nodes	Anterior: Sterno-hyoid muscle's lateral border. Posterior: Sternocleidomastoid muscle's posterior border. Superior: Hyoid bone. Inferior: Cricoid notch (clinical), omohyoid muscle (surgical)		Internal jugular vein, carotid arteries

(continued)

Table 1.1 (continued)

Level	Name	Boundaries (anatomical)	Subdivisions and notes	Key structures
IV	Lower jugular nodes	Anterior: Sterno-hyoid muscle's lateral border. Posterior: Sternocleidomastoid muscle's posterior border. Superior: Cricoid notch (clinical), omohyoid muscle (surgical). Inferior: Clavicle		Internal jugular vein, subclavian artery, thoracic duct (left side)
V	Posterior triangle	Anterior: Sternocleidomastoid muscle's posterior border. Posterior: Trapezius muscle's anterior border. Inferior: Clavicle	Subdivided into VA (superiorly) and VB (inferiorly) separated by a horizontal plane marking the inferior border of the anterior cricoid arch; VA contains spinal accessory lymph nodes, VB contains transverse cervical nodes and supraclavicular nodes	Spinal accessory nerve, cervical plexus, brachial plexus
VI	Anterior compartment nodes	Lateral: Sterno-hyoid muscle's lateral border. Superior: Hyoid bone. Inferior: Suprasternal notch	Contains pretracheal, paratracheal, precricoid lymph nodes	Thyroid gland, parathyroid glands, recurrent laryngeal nerve, trachea

in patients with high-risk features, such as extranodal extension, positive surgical margins, or advanced nodal disease. PET/CT is used for surveillance of disease.

1.4 Submandibular Gland Excision

Indications for Surgery [10]

- Benign or malignant tumours of the submandibular gland
- Recurrent sialadenitis or sialolithiasis not responding to conservative management
- Asymptomatic, enlarging submandibular gland masses
- Diagnosis of a suspicious lesion when fine-needle aspiration cytology is inconclusive
- As part of level I neck dissection

Specific Risks Involved with the Surgery

- Neural structure injury to the marginal mandibular branch of the facial nerve, lingual nerve, or hypoglossal nerve injury
- Haematoma
- Infection
- Sialocele or salivary fistula

Steps of the Surgery

1. Administer general anaesthesia and endotracheal intubation.
2. Position the patient supine, with the head turned away from the side to be operated on stabilized in a head ring and the neck extended with a shoulder roll.
3. Consider facial nerve monitoring.
4. Mark the incision line 2–3 cm below the lower border of the mandible, extending from the angle of the mandible to the midline (Fig. 1.7). This reduces the chance of injury to the marginal mandibular nerve.
5. Consider injecting local anaesthetic such as Lignospan (1:80,000 adrenaline) or 1:100,000 pure adrenaline for haemostasis.
6. Make a skin incision along the marked line, and carefully develop subplatysmal flaps superiorly and inferiorly.
7. Identify the facial vein, and ligate it for better exposure of the submandibular gland and surrounding structures.
8. Carefully identify and preserve the marginal mandibular branch of the facial nerve during dissection by using the Hayes-Martin manoeuvre which entails ligation of the posterior facial vein and reflection of the fascia upwards to preserve the marginal mandibular nerve (which lies within this fascia).
9. Dissect the gland off the underlying mylohyoid muscle, starting from the posterior border and proceeding anteriorly.
10. Dissect the gland free from the floor of the mouth and the submandibular duct (Wharton's duct), ligating the duct as needed.
11. Achieve haemostasis, and inspect the surgical field.
12. Close the wound in layers using appropriate sutures, and place a drain if necessary.

Important Points to Note During the Surgery

- Adequate exposure of the surgical field is essential for a successful procedure.
- Preserve the marginal mandibular branch of the facial nerve by carefully identifying it and avoiding injury to the nerve during dissection. An appreciation of the anatomy is key, as seen in Figs. 1.6 and 1.7. Alternatively, perform the Hayes-Martin manoeuvre to safely dissect the gland deeper to the nerve.

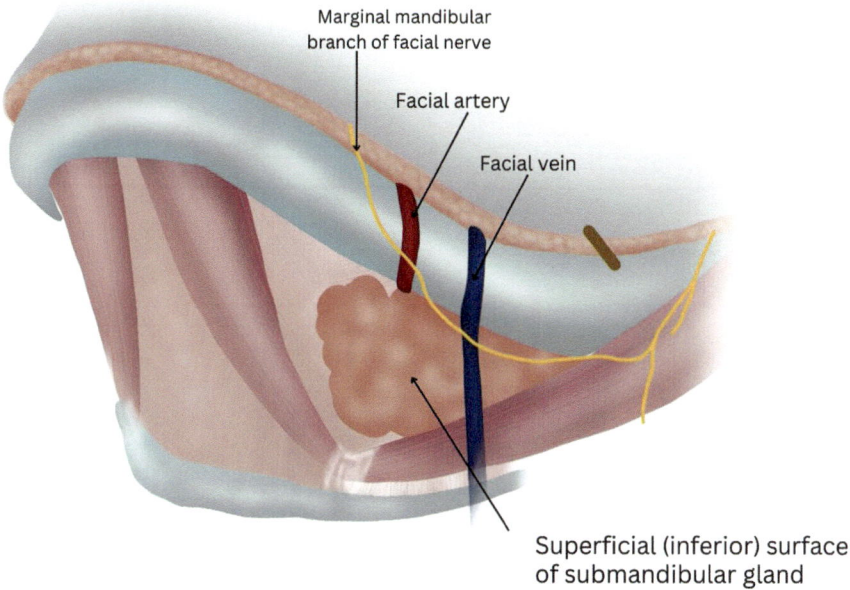

Fig. 1.6 Anatomy of the submandibular gland. Illustrated by Vikum Liyanaarachchi

- Meticulous haemostasis is crucial to prevent post-operative haematoma and complications.

Questions a Consultant Might Ask a Trainee About the Operation

1. **Can you describe the anatomical relationship between the submandibular gland, the facial artery and vein, and the marginal mandibular branch of the facial nerve?**
   The submandibular gland is situated in the submandibular triangle, bordered by the mandible's lower edge, the anterior and posterior bellies of the digastric muscle, and the stylohyoid muscle [11]. The facial artery and vein are found medial to the gland, crossing over the posterior belly of the digastric muscle. The marginal mandibular branch of the facial nerve runs parallel to the lower border of the mandible, crossing superficial to the facial artery and vein.
2. **How do you differentiate between benign and malignant lesions of the submandibular gland intraoperatively?**
   Intraoperative assessment of submandibular gland lesions can be challenging, as benign and malignant lesions may have similar appearances. Factors that suggest malignancy include irregular borders, invasion of adjacent structures, and

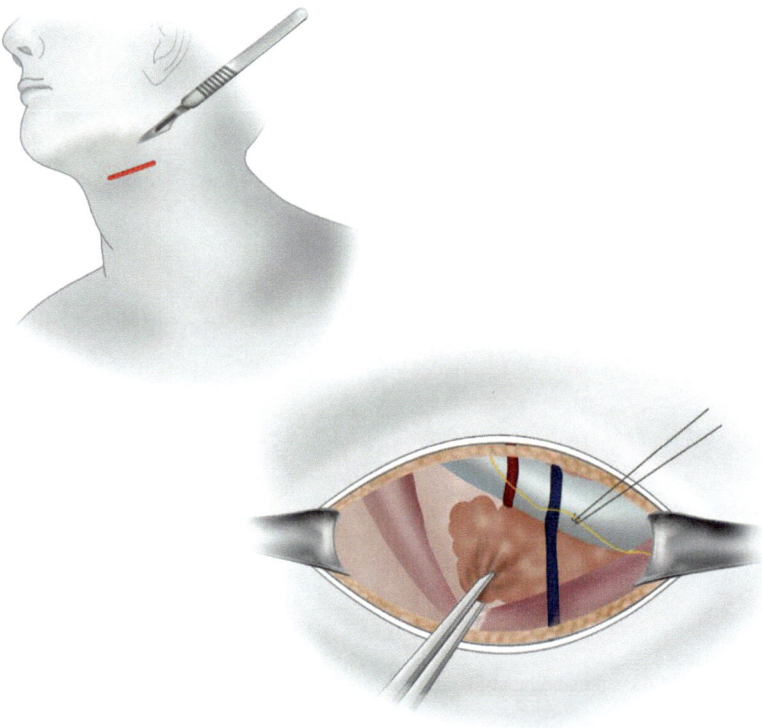

Fig. 1.7 Incision made 2 cm below mandible to avoid marginal mandibular nerve injury. Illustrated by Vikum Liyanaarachchi

presence of enlarged or abnormal lymph nodes. Frozen section analysis can be helpful in differentiating benign from malignant lesions during surgery.
3. **What steps can be taken to minimize the risk of injury to the marginal mandibular branch of the facial nerve during the procedure?**
    - Understanding the nerve's anatomy [11]: The marginal mandibular branch of the facial nerve is responsible for motor innervation to the muscles of the lower lip and chin. It typically runs just below the mandible, often within 1–2 cm below the lower border, and is more superficial where it crosses the facial artery. The nerve can be at risk during surgeries involving the lower face, particularly in the area ranging from the angle of the mandible to the symphysis.
    - Use of the Hayes-Martin manoeuvre: The Hayes-Martin manoeuvre involves the ligation and division of the posterior facial vein, which helps in providing better access and visibility to the marginal mandibular nerve as it runs beneath

the mandible. By doing so, this manoeuvre facilitates the superior reflection of the investing layer of the deep cervical fascia. This reflection is done carefully below the mandible, which not only exposes but also helps to protect the marginal mandibular branch of the facial nerve by moving it away from the surgical field where dissections are being performed. This approach is particularly useful in neck dissections and other surgeries in the submandibular region to avoid inadvertent nerve damage.
- Staying superficial and close to the gland: When performing dissection near the submandibular gland, it is important to stay superficial and close to the glandular tissue. This practice helps in avoiding deeper dissections where the nerve could potentially be located.
- Intraoperative nerve monitoring: Utilizing nerve monitoring can be an effective way to identify and preserve the facial nerve's branches during surgery. This technology provides real-time feedback and can alert the surgical team if the nerve's integrity is at risk.
- Use of magnification: Loupes or operative microscopes enhance the surgeon's ability to see smaller structures like nerves and can significantly contribute to safer dissection.

4. **How would you manage a post-operative sialocele or salivary fistula?**

   Post-operative sialocele or salivary fistula management depends on the severity and duration of the condition. In general, conservative measures including pressure dressings, anti-sialagogue medications, and aspiration of the sialocele are enough. If conservative measures fail or the fistula persists, surgical intervention may be necessary, such as fistula closure, sialocele marsupialization, or placement of a sclerosing agent.

5. **What is the relationship between the lingual nerve and the submandibular duct?**

   The relationship between the lingual nerve and the submandibular duct (also known as Wharton's duct) is characterized by a distinctive triple relationship. Initially, the lingual nerve passes lateral to the submandibular duct. As it continues its course, it then loops inferiorly around the duct. Finally, the nerve crosses to the medial side of the duct. This anatomical configuration is important for surgical and diagnostic procedures in the oral and submandibular regions, as it presents a potential risk area for nerve damage during operations involving the submandibular gland and its duct.

6. **What is the effect of marginal mandibular nerve (MMN) injury?**

   The marginal mandibular nerve (MMN) innervates several facial muscles, primarily the depressor anguli oris and depressor labii inferioris. Injury to this nerve can lead to paralysis of these muscles, which results in the upward rotation of the ipsilateral angle of the mouth. This occurs because the unopposed action of the levator labii superioris muscle causes an upward pull. The patient typically exhibits an asymmetry in the lower face, specifically characterized by a drooping of the lower lip on the affected side.

7. **What is the nerve supply of the submandibular gland?**

The innervation of the submandibular gland involves both parasympathetic and sympathetic nervous systems, each contributing to its function in different ways [11]:

Parasympathetic Innervation: Preganglionic fibres of the parasympathetic nervous system travel through the chorda tympani, a branch of the facial nerve. These fibres reach the submandibular ganglion, where they synapse. The postganglionic fibres then emerge from the submandibular ganglion and join the lingual nerve. These fibres are responsible for stimulating the submandibular gland to produce saliva, a crucial function for digestion and oral health.

Sympathetic innervation: The sympathetic innervation of the submandibular gland involves postganglionic fibres originating from the superior cervical ganglion. These fibres travel along the branches of the external carotid artery (ECA) to reach the submandibular gland. The sympathetic nervous system primarily modulates the gland's blood flow and can slightly alter saliva production, generally reducing it during sympathetic activation (e.g. stress conditions).

1.5 Parotidectomy

Indications for Surgery [12]

- Benign or malignant tumours of the parotid gland
- Recurrent parotitis not responding to conservative management
- Diagnosis of a suspicious lesion when fine-needle aspiration cytology is inconclusive
- Parotid gland involvement in autoimmune disorders, such as Sjögren's syndrome, requiring tissue diagnosis

Specific Risks Involved with the Surgery

- Injury to the facial nerve (FN): transient dysfunction (up to 50%), permanent dysfunction
- Haematoma
- Infection
- Salivary fistula or sialocele
- Frey's syndrome
- Numbness to ear lobe + wound site (injury to GAN)
- First bite syndrome (if deep lobe of parotid was excised)
- Cosmetic change of the contour of the face

Steps of the Surgery

1. Administer general anaesthesia and endotracheal intubation.
2. Position the patient supine, with the head turned away stabilized in a head ring from the side to be operated on and the neck extended with a shoulder roll.
3. Place the leads for a two- or four-channel facial nerve monitor intraoperatively.
4. Mark the incision line: preauricular incision extending around the earlobe and down the posterior hairline (modified Blair incision) or along the natural skin crease in the neck (Fig. 1.8).
5. Consider injecting local anaesthetic such as Lignospan (1:80,000 adrenaline) or 1:100,000 pure adrenaline for haemostasis.
6. Make a skin incision along the marked line, and develop sub-superficial muscular aponeurotic system (SMAS) flaps anteriorly +/− posteriorly. Or find the platysma at the anterior/inferior aspect of your incision, and work towards the top end.
7. Identify the parotid gland, and divide the superficial fascia overlying the gland.
8. Identify and dissect the anterior boarder of SCM, and then find the posterior digastric muscle (deep landmark for FN), tragal pointer, and tympano-mastoid suture (Fig. 1.9).

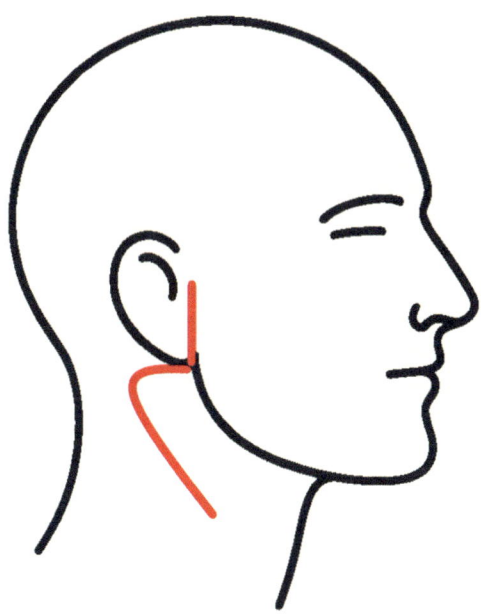

Fig. 1.8 Modified Blair incision for parotidectomy

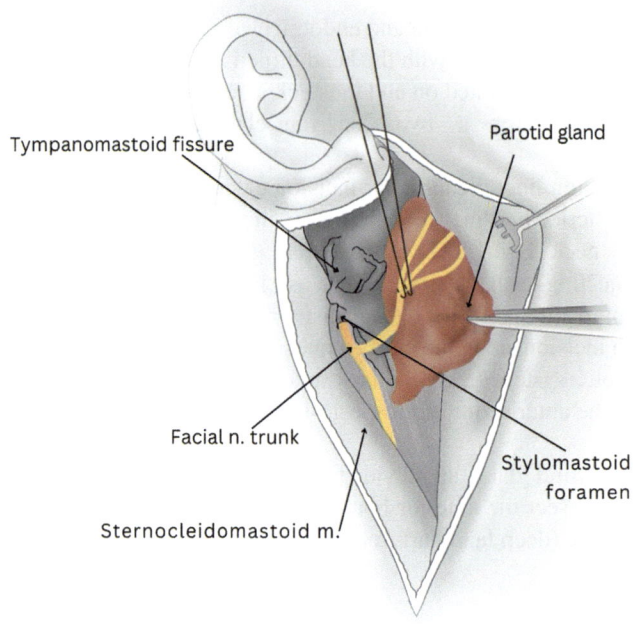

Fig. 1.9 Facial nerve in relation to tympanomastoid suture. Illustrated by Vikum Liyanaarachchi

9. Identify the main trunk of the facial nerve at the stylomastoid foramen or using a nerve stimulator, and then trace its branches through the gland. This requires time and patience.
10. Avoid tunnelling, and achieve wide-field exposure for dissection of the gland.
11. Perform a superficial or total parotidectomy, depending on the extent of the disease, while preserving the facial nerve branches.
12. Remove the tumour and surrounding parotid tissue en bloc, ensuring clear margins.
13. Achieve haemostasis, and inspect the surgical field.
14. Close the wound in layers using appropriate sutures, and place a drain if necessary.

Important Points to Note During the Surgery

- Adequate exposure of the surgical field and identification of the facial nerve are crucial for a successful procedure.

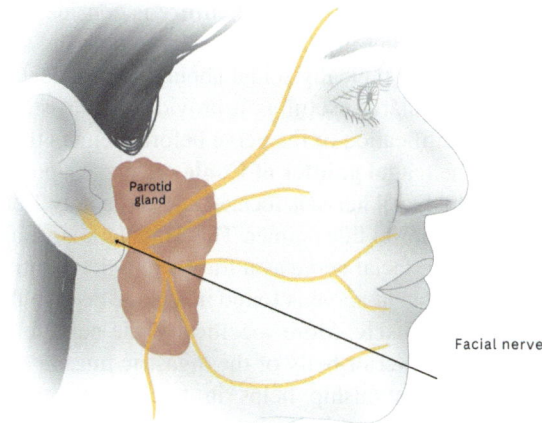

Fig. 1.10 Facial nerve anatomy through the parotid gland. Illustrated by Vikum Liyanaarachchi

- Preserve the facial nerve branches by carefully identifying and avoiding injury to the nerve during dissection (Fig. 1.10).
- Meticulous haemostasis is essential to prevent post-operative haematoma and complications.

Questions a Consultant Might Ask a Trainee During the Operation

1. **What are the indications for parotidectomy, and what preoperative investigations are necessary to evaluate these cases?**

    Indications for parotidectomy include benign or malignant tumours, recurrent parotitis not responding to conservative management, inconclusive fine-needle aspiration cytology results, and parotid gland involvement in autoimmune disorders requiring tissue diagnosis [12]. Preoperative investigations may include ultrasound, computed tomography (CT), magnetic resonance imaging (MRI), and fine-needle aspiration cytology to assess the lesion's nature and extent.

2. **Can you describe the anatomical relationship between the parotid gland and the facial nerve?**

    The parotid gland is situated in the preauricular region, superficial to the ramus of the mandible. The facial nerve (cranial nerve VII) enters the gland at its posteromedial aspect after exiting the stylomastoid foramen [13]. Within the gland, the facial nerve divides into two main divisions, the temporofacial and cervicofacial branches, which further divide into multiple branches, supplying the muscles of facial expression.

3. **What are the facial nerve landmarks during parotidectomy surgery [13]?**
   - The **tympano-mastoid suture** is considered the most reliable landmark for identifying the facial nerve as it exits the stylomastoid foramen. The facial nerve is typically found about 3–6 mm deep to this suture. This landmark is particularly useful as it provides a consistent reference point for the initial identification of the nerve before it enters the parotid gland.
   - The **tragal pointer of Conley** refers to a point near the cartilage of the tragus. The facial nerve is located approximately 1 cm deep, 1 cm inferior, and 1 cm anterior to this pointer. This landmark is valuable for locating the main trunk of the facial nerve as it travels into the parotid gland.
   - The facial nerve is found in a plane deep to the **posterior belly of the digastric muscle**. More specifically, the nerve bisects the angle formed between the posterior belly of the digastric muscle and the skull base. This anatomical relationship helps in tracking the nerve as it branches within the parotid gland.
   - Although not as precise as the tympano-mastoid suture or the tragal pointer, the **angle of the mandible** serves as a general guide to the lateral boundary of where the facial nerve can be located.
   - The **retromandibular vein**, often found within the parotid gland, can serve as an additional guide. The vein typically lies posterior to the facial nerve, and its identification can help suggest the location of the facial nerve branches.
4. **What other options are available if there is difficulty in finding the pes anserinus or a tumour is overlying the facial nerve trunk?**

   When encountering difficulty in locating the facial nerve or when a tumour is overlying the facial nerve trunk during surgical procedures, several alternative strategies can be employed to ensure safe and effective identification and preservation of the nerve:

   Retrograde approach:
   - Employing a retrograde technique by identifying distal branches of the facial nerve and tracing them back to the main trunk can be an effective method. This approach is particularly useful in complex cases where direct access to the nerve trunk is obstructed. It helps in avoiding accidental nerve damage by providing a clearer path of dissection.

   Nerve monitoring:
   - Utilizing intraoperative nerve monitoring provides real-time feedback on the functionality of the facial nerve during surgery. This technology enhances the surgeon's ability to detect the nerve's location and activity, thereby reducing the risk of unintentional injury.

   Refinement of anatomical landmarks:
   - Marginal mandibular nerve: This branch generally lies approximately 1–1.5 cm below the angle of the mandible. Identifying this landmark can guide surgeons in safely navigating the lower facial regions.
   - Buccal branch: Often found about 1 cm below the parotid duct. The parotid (Stensen's) duct itself can be located along the middle third of a line stretching

from the midpoint of the external auditory canal to a point midway between the nasal ala and the angle of the mouth.
   - Zygomatic branch: Typically located about 1 cm below the midpoint between the lateral canthus and the tragus, pinpointing this branch can help map the course of the upper facial branches.
5. **What steps should be taken in case of an intraoperative capsular breach of a pleomorphic adenoma?**
   - Prevent further spillage by suturing the breach or holding it with gauze.
   - Thoroughly irrigate the tumour bed with warmed saline at the end of the operation.
   - Discuss the case in a multidisciplinary team (MDT) meeting to consider radiotherapy, considering the patient's age, comorbidities, preferences, and degree of concern about microscopic residual disease.
6. **What are the different surgical approaches to access the deep lobe of the parotid gland?**
   - Trans-parotid approach
   - Trans-cervical or trans-cervical-trans-parotid approach, especially if the tumour extends into the parapharyngeal space
   - Trans-mandibular approach
   - Transoral robotic surgical approach
7. **When should neck dissection be considered in cases of parotid malignancy?**
   According to the ENT UK Guidelines 2016 [14, 15]:
   - For N0 (no regional lymph node metastasis): Elective selective neck dissection (SND) of levels I–III is recommended if the cancer is high stage or clinically high grade. Some will consider level Va.
   - For N+ (presence of regional lymph node metastasis): Perform a therapeutic neck dissection.
   - As a general rule, neck dissection is recommended for all parotid malignancies except for small, low-grade cancers.
8. **What are the different types of parotidectomy?**
   There are several types of parotidectomy, which can be categorized based on the extent of gland removal and preservation of the facial nerve. The main types of parotidectomy include the following [12]:
   - **Extracapsular** dissection: This procedure involves the removal of a parotid gland tumour along with a thin layer of normal parotid tissue around the tumour. It is typically performed for small, benign tumours located in the superficial lobe of the gland and is associated with lower rates of facial nerve injury.
   - **Superficial** parotidectomy: This is the most common type of parotidectomy and involves the removal of the superficial lobe of the parotid gland. The facial nerve is identified and preserved during the procedure. Superficial parotidectomy is used for benign and malignant tumours located in the superficial lobe of the gland.

- **Total** parotidectomy: This procedure involves the removal of the entire parotid gland, including both the superficial and deep lobes. The facial nerve is identified and preserved during the operation. Total parotidectomy is performed for malignant tumours or large, deep-seated benign tumours.
- **Radical** parotidectomy: This procedure is similar to a total parotidectomy, but it also involves the removal of adjacent structures, such as the facial nerve, lymph nodes, or other tissues infiltrated by a malignant tumour. Reconstruction of the facial nerve may be required following this procedure.
- **Modified radical** parotidectomy: This procedure involves the removal of the entire parotid gland as well as the resection of additional structures (e.g. lymph nodes or adjacent soft tissue) that may be involved by the tumour. However, unlike radical parotidectomy, the facial nerve is preserved in a modified radical parotidectomy.

1.6 Laryngectomy (Total, Partial, Supraglottic)

Indications for Surgery [16]

- Advanced laryngeal cancer not amenable to organ preservation therapy
- Recurrent laryngeal cancer after radiation or chemoradiation therapy
- Persistent aspiration or airway obstruction due to laryngeal dysfunction
- Severe laryngeal trauma

Specific Risks Involved with the Surgery [16]

- Haemorrhage
- Infection
- Pharyngocutaneous fistula
- Dysphagia
- Aspiration in partial laryngectomy
- Recurrent chest infections in partial laryngectomy
- Hypothyroidism
- Hypoparathyroidism and hypocalcaemia
- Permanent tracheostomy: 100% (after total laryngectomy)
- Loss of voice and smell (after total laryngectomy)
- Chyle leak (mostly in total and partial laryngectomies)
- Hypoglossal nerve injury
- Marginal mandibular nerve palsy

Steps of the Surgery (Total Laryngectomy)

1. Administer general anaesthesia, and perform oral/nasal intubation or tracheotomy, depending on the airway's condition.

1 Head and Neck

2. Position the patient supine in a head ring with the neck extended using a shoulder roll.
3. Consider injecting local anaesthetic such as Lignospan (1:80,000 adrenaline) or 1:100,000 adrenaline for haemostasis.
4. Make a Gluck-Sorenson incision (long apron) as seen in Fig. 1.11 or short apron if narrow-field laryngectomy.
5. Develop subplatysmal flaps superiorly and inferiorly.
6. Identify the SCMs, and divide the sternal head of the muscle to avoid narrow, deep stoma.
7. Divide the strap muscles including omohyoid muscle, and retract them superiorly to expose the larynx and trachea.
8. Identify and ligate the superior and middle thyroid vessels.
9. Consider incorporating the ipsilateral hemithyroid to the tumour for oncological clearance.
10. Transect the pharynx (suprahyoid pharyngotomy) circumferentially above the level of the larynx with caution at greater cornu of hyoid bone to avoid injury of hypoglossal nerve.
11. Divide the trachea below the level of the tumour, and remove the larynx en bloc.
12. Perform cricopharyngeal myotomy to improve the vibration of pharyngo-oesophageal segment for better voicing.
13. Perform a primary tracheoesophageal puncture for voice prosthesis placement if desired.
14. Insert nasogastric tube for feeding.
15. Consider inserting salivary bypass tube, particularly in salvage laryngectomy.
16. Close the pharyngeal mucosa with absorbable sutures.
17. Create a tracheostoma, and suture the trachea to the skin.
18. Close the platysma and skin in layers, and place a drain if necessary.

Important Points to Note During the Surgery

- Adequate exposure of the larynx and surrounding structures is crucial for a successful procedure.
- Meticulous haemostasis is essential to prevent post-operative haematoma and complications.
- Preserve as much functional laryngeal tissue as possible to maintain voice and swallowing function.
- Make sure that the patient receives tracheostomy training as airway is now through stoma in the neck as seen in Fig. 1.12.

Questions a Consultant Might Ask a Trainee During the Operation

1. **What are the indications for different types of laryngectomies, and what preoperative investigations are necessary to evaluate these cases?**

Fig. 1.11 Gluck-Sorenson (long apron) incision (front and side views)

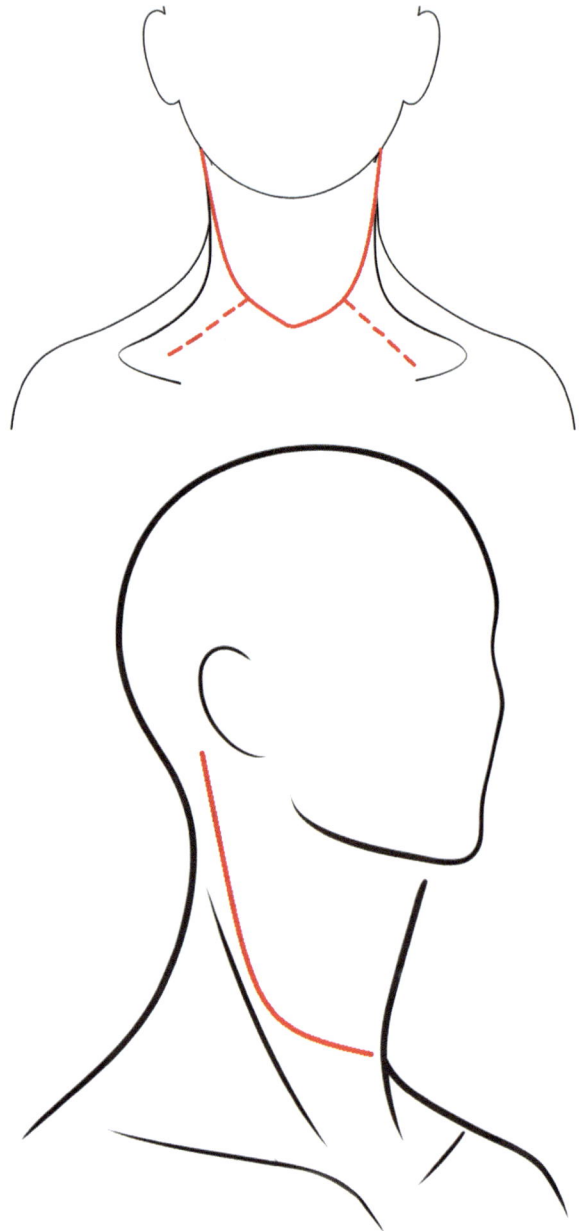

Indications for different types of laryngectomy include advanced laryngeal cancer not amenable to organ preservation therapy, recurrent laryngeal cancer after radiation or chemoradiation therapy, persistent aspiration or airway obstruction due to laryngeal dysfunction, and severe laryngeal trauma [16]. Preoperative

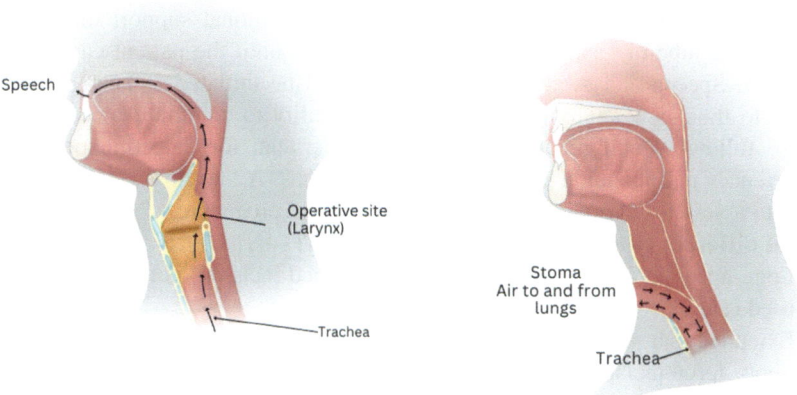

Fig. 1.12 Laryngectomy before and after

investigations may include computed tomography (CT), magnetic resonance imaging (MRI), positron emission tomography (PET), and endoscopy to assess the tumour's nature and extent, as well as preoperative speech and language therapy assessment and pulmonary function tests to evaluate the patient's respiratory status.

2. **Can you describe the anatomical structures involved in each type of laryngectomy?**

    The anatomical structures involved in each type of laryngectomy vary based on the extent of the surgery. In total laryngectomy, the entire larynx, including the epiglottis, true and false vocal cords, cricoid cartilage, and arytenoids, is removed (Fig. 1.11). In partial laryngectomy, a portion of the larynx is removed depending on the tumour's location and extent, preserving a functional laryngeal remnant. In supraglottic laryngectomy, the supraglottic structures, including the epiglottis, false vocal cords, aryepiglottic folds, and arytenoids, can be removed, while the true vocal cords and other laryngeal structures are preserved [16].

3. **What are the key steps in performing a primary tracheoesophageal puncture for voice prosthesis placement during total laryngectomy?**

    Performing a primary tracheoesophageal puncture for voice prosthesis placement during total laryngectomy involves creating a small hole between the posterior tracheal wall and the anterior oesophageal wall after the larynx has been removed. This puncture is typically made at the level of the second or third tracheal ring. A voice prosthesis (one-way valve) is then inserted through the puncture, connecting the trachea and the oesophagus to allow for post-operative voice restoration.

4. **What are the post-operative considerations for patients undergoing laryngectomy, and how do you manage potential complications?**

Post-operative considerations for patients undergoing laryngectomy include monitoring for complications such as haemorrhage, infection, pharyngocutaneous fistula, dysphagia, and chyle leak. Regular wound assessment, drain management, and tracheostomy care are essential. Nutritional support through a nasogastric tube or gastrostomy may be necessary until the patient can safely swallow. Speech and swallowing therapy should be initiated to help patients adapt to their new anatomy and regain their ability to communicate and eat. Close follow-up and regular surveillance are crucial for detecting potential recurrences and managing long-term complications. A barium swallow test is used to assess for leaks a few days after the surgical procedure.

5. **What different types of laryngectomy incisions?**
   - Long-apron incision (Gluck-Sorenson U-shaped incision) is the commonest used [16].
   - Extended long-apron incision if neck dissection is planned.
   - Short-apron incision with separate stoma (better cosmesis, but limited exposure of lower neck).
   - Other incisions are rarely used: as T, horizontal double-Y incision, or trap-door incision.

6. **What are the operative steps to improve the quality of voice rehabilitation?**
   - Tension-free (and if possible) horizontal closure of the pharynx
   - Upper oesophageal myotomy
   - Pharyngeal plexus neurectomy
   - Primary puncture, if possible, especially if not a salvage laryngectomy
   - Division of the sternal heads of sternomastoid leading to a flattening of the lower neck, which aids stomal dressing adhesion and humidity and moisture exchanger (HME) fixation

7. **What is the minimum width of pharyngeal remnant that allows for primary closure?**

   For successful primary closure of a pharyngeal remnant, preservation of the mucosa of at least one pyriform fossa is required, which typically measures around 1.5 cm in a relaxed state and can extend up to 2.5 cm when stretched. If the remaining pharyngeal width is less than this, considering a flap reconstruction is advisable to ensure adequate closure and function.

8. **What types of pharyngeal mucosal closures are used in laryngectomy:**

   In laryngectomy surgeries, pharyngeal mucosal closures are crucial to ensure a secure and functional post-operative outcome. Here is an expanded explanation of the two primary techniques used for mucosal closures in laryngectomy—the modified Connell and Lambert techniques:

   Modified Connell technique:
   - Description: This technique involves a continuous, interlocking suture pattern that is primarily used to minimize tension across the suture line. The interlocking nature of the stitch helps distribute the tension evenly along the length of the closure.

- Advantages: The reduced tension decreases the risk of tearing and wound stress, potentially lowering the chance of post-operative complications like leakage.
- Risks: The major drawback is that if the continuous suture knot fails or breaks, there is a risk of the entire suture line coming undone, leading to wound dehiscence (reopening of the closed wound).
- Application: Intraluminal sutures are placed and are inverted to enhance the healing by placing the knot inside the lumen, thus minimizing exposure to external factors that could interfere with the wound healing.
  Lambert technique:
- Description: This technique uses interrupted sutures, which means that each stitch is individually knotted.
- Advantages: Interrupted sutures are generally more secure than a continuous suture line because if one suture fails, the rest remain intact, thus localizing any potential dehiscence.
- Disadvantages: The primary disadvantage is that each suture individually bears more tension than in an interlocking continuous suture. This increased tension can lead to greater stress at each suture point, which might compromise the wound integrity or delay healing.
- Application: The stitches are placed extra-mucosally and are also inverted. By placing the stitches outside the mucosal layer, there is less disturbance to the mucosa itself, potentially promoting better healing while the inverted stitches help in creating a smoother internal surface and reducing the risk of granulation tissue formation.

9. **What is a narrow-field laryngectomy?**

    A narrow-field laryngectomy is a surgical approach designed as a less invasive alternative to a total laryngectomy. It is particularly utilized for patients suffering from intractable aspiration, where other less invasive measures have failed to improve their condition.

    The key features of this procedure:
    - Muscle preservation: Unlike in a total laryngectomy, the narrow-field laryngectomy aims to spare the strap muscles, which are important for neck structure and function. Preserving these muscles helps in reducing post-operative morbidity and aids in a quicker recovery.
    - High tracheal transection: This technique involves transecting the trachea at a higher level than in a standard laryngectomy. This strategic cut minimizes the amount of tracheal tissue removed and aims to maintain better structural and functional integrity in the neck.
    - Conservation of pharyngeal mucosa: A critical aspect of this procedure is preserving as much pharyngeal mucosa as possible. This is essential for maintaining swallowing function post-surgery. In some cases, even the mucosa covering the epiglottis may be preserved to reduce the pharyngeal opening further, which helps in managing aspiration by limiting the entry of food or liquid into the lower respiratory tract.

- Reduced pharyngeal opening: By creating a smaller pharyngeal opening, the procedure reduces the risk of aspiration, which is the primary goal in patients for whom the surgery is indicated.

1.7 Excision of Branchial Cleft Cysts

Indications for Surgery [17]

- Branchial cleft cyst causing symptoms or infection
- Cosmetic concerns
- Aspiration or biopsy indicating potential malignancy
- Recurrent infections

Specific Risks Involved with the Surgery

- Haemorrhage
- Infection
- Recurrence of the cyst
- Injury to adjacent structures, such as nerves (marginal mandibular nerve, hypoglossal and spinal accessory nerve), vessels (internal jugular vein), and parotid gland
- Scarring

Steps of the Surgery

1. Administer general anaesthesia, and perform endotracheal intubation.
2. Position the patient supine, with the head turned away stabilized in a head ring from the side to be operated on and the neck extended with a shoulder roll.
3. Identify the location of the branchial cleft cyst and its relationship to surrounding structures.
4. Consider injecting local anaesthetic such as Lignospan (1:80,000 adrenaline) or 1:100,000 adrenaline for haemostasis.
5. Make an elliptical skin incision around the cyst, incorporating the previous drainage site (if applicable).
6. Dissect the cyst meticulously from the surrounding tissues, staying close to the cyst, preserving vital structures such as nerves and vessels.
7. Trace the tract of the cyst, if present, and excise it in its entirety.
8. Remove the cyst en bloc, ensuring that the entire cyst wall is excised to minimize the risk of recurrence.
9. Achieve meticulous haemostasis to prevent post-operative haematoma formation.
10. Place a drain if necessary

11. Close the wound in layers using absorbable sutures for deep tissue and non-absorbable sutures or staples for the skin.
12. Apply a sterile dressing.

Important Points to Note During the Surgery

- Careful dissection close to the cyst and preservation of vital structures are crucial to avoid complications.
- Complete excision of the cyst and its tract is essential to minimize the risk of recurrence.
- Meticulous haemostasis is important to prevent post-operative haematoma formation.
- A good understanding of the anatomical course is seen in Fig. 1.13.

Questions a Consultant Might Ask a Trainee During the Operation

1. **Can you describe the embryological origin and classification of branchial cleft anomalies?**
   Branchial cleft anomalies arise from incomplete obliteration of the branchial clefts and pouches during embryologic development. They can be classified into four types based on their origin: first branchial cleft cysts (type I and type II), second branchial cleft cysts, third branchial cleft cysts, and fourth branchial cleft cysts. First branchial cleft cysts are the most common, accounting for 90% of cases [17].
2. **What are the potential differential diagnoses for a neck mass in this location, and how can they be differentiated preoperatively?**
   Potential differential diagnoses for a neck mass in the location of a branchial cleft cyst include lymphadenopathy, lipoma, sebaceous cyst, dermoid cyst, thyroglossal duct cyst, and metastatic lymph nodes. A thorough history, physical examination, and imaging studies, such as ultrasound, computed tomography (CT), magnetic resonance imaging (MRI), or positron emission tomography (PET)/CT, can help differentiate these entities preoperatively. Fine-needle aspiration (FNA) biopsy may also be used for further evaluation.
3. **What imaging studies are helpful in evaluating a suspected branchial cleft cyst?**
   Imaging studies helpful in evaluating a suspected branchial cleft cyst include ultrasound, CT, and MRI. Ultrasound can be useful for assessing the cyst's size, location, and relationship to adjacent structures. CT, MRI, and PET/CT provide more detailed information about the cyst and its tract, as well as the relationship to surrounding tissues, and can help differentiate a branchial cleft cyst from other neck masses depending on its FDG avidity.
4. **How do you manage a branchial cleft cyst that has become infected prior to surgery?**

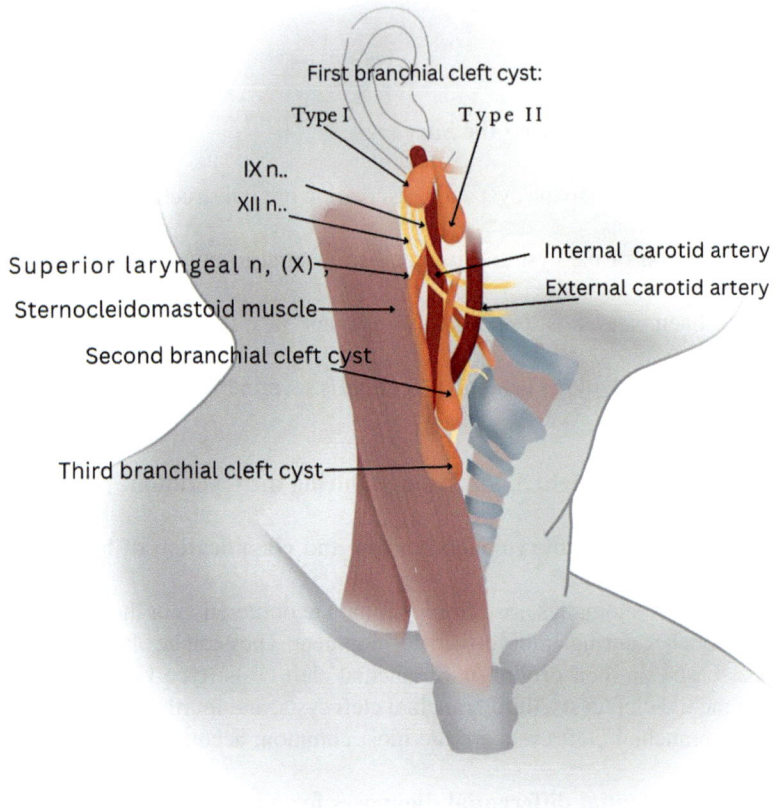

Fig. 1.13 Branchial cleft cysts shown in relation to other structures in the neck (first, second, and third cleft cysts). Illustrated by Vikum Liyanaarachchi

If a branchial cleft cyst has become infected prior to surgery, initial management should focus on controlling the infection. This may involve antibiotic therapy, incision, and drainage if an abscess has formed, and close monitoring for complications. Once the infection has been adequately controlled, definitive surgical excision can be planned.

5. **What is the anatomical/operative course of the second branchial cleft tract?**

    The anatomical and operative course of the second branchial cleft tract is a key consideration in the diagnosis and surgical management of related congenital anomalies. These anomalies typically follow a well-defined path, which reflects their embryonic origin from the second branchial cleft.
    - External opening: The external opening of the tract is typically located along the anterior border of the neck. It often appears along the carotid sheath, situ-

ated between the external and internal carotid arteries. This superficial location makes it visible and palpable upon clinical examination.
- Course relative to cranial nerves: The tract courses superficially relative to cranial nerve XII (the hypoglossal nerve) and cranial nerve IX (the glossopharyngeal nerve). This relationship is crucial for surgical planning to avoid nerve damage. The tract's proximity to these nerves demands careful dissection and monitoring during surgical intervention.
- Internal opening: The internal opening of the tract can be found at the level of the middle constrictor muscle of the pharynx or within the tonsillar fossa. This ending point reflects the deep penetration of the tract, which can have implications for the spread of infection and the complexity of surgical management.

6. **What are the anatomical variations of branchial cleft cyst?**
   Bailey Classification of Branchial Cleft Cysts [18]:
   - Type I: Located deep to the platysma and anterior to the sternocleidomastoid (SCM) muscle. It is the second most common type of branchial cleft cyst and typically presents as a mass that does not move with swallowing or protrusion of the tongue.
   - Type II: Characterized by its proximity to the internal carotid artery and its adherence to the internal jugular vein. This is the most common type and poses a significant risk during surgical removal due to its close relationship with major vascular structures.
   - Type III: Extends between the internal and external carotid arteries, which can complicate surgical access and requires careful planning to avoid vascular injury.
   - Type IV: Abuts the pharyngeal wall and may extend superiorly to the skull base. This type can be particularly challenging to manage due to its potential involvement with critical deep structures of the neck and skull base.

7. **What is the investigation of choice in third or fourth branchial cleft anomalies?**
   The investigation of choice for third or fourth branchial cleft anomalies is typically a barium swallow. This imaging study helps in delineating the presence of any fistulous tract or cyst that communicates with the pharyngeal or oesophageal lumen, thus aiding in diagnosis and surgical planning.

8. **What is the management of third and fourth branchial cleft anomalies?**
   Surgical excision: Complete surgical excision of the cyst or fistula is necessary to prevent recurrence. For third and fourth branchial cleft anomalies, this typically includes an ipsilateral partial thyroidectomy, as these anomalies often have tracts that pass close to or through thyroid tissue. This approach ensures that any potential thyroid involvement is addressed.

   Endoscopic approaches: For less invasive management or when surgical risks are considered high, endoscopic obliteration may be employed. This technique involves the use of diathermy to cauterize the tract and the application of tissue glue to seal the piriform opening. This method can be an effective alternative, particularly for small fistulas or for patients with significant comorbidities.

1.8 Thyroglossal Duct Cyst Excision (Modified Sistrunk Procedure)

Indications for Surgery [19]

- Recurrent or persistent thyroglossal duct cyst
- History of duct infection or abscess formation
- Mass effect
- Suspicion of malignancy (potential risk of <1% transformation into papillary thyroid cancer)
- Cosmetic concerns

Specific Risks Involved with the Surgery [19]

- Haemorrhage
- Infection
- Recurrence of the cyst
- Injury to the adjacent structures (e.g. hypoglossal nerve, blood vessels)
- Hypothyroidism (if a significant portion of the thyroid gland is removed)

Steps of the Surgery

1. Administer general anaesthesia, and perform endotracheal intubation.
2. Position the patient supine, with the head supported on a head ring with the neck extended using a shoulder roll.
3. Identify the location of the thyroglossal duct cyst and its relationship to the hyoid bone and thyroid gland.
4. Consider injecting local anaesthetic such as Lignospan (1:80,000 adrenaline) or 1:100,000 adrenaline for haemostasis.
5. Make a horizontal skin incision over the cyst, ideally in a skin crease.
6. Dissect subplatysmal flaps to expose the cyst and the surrounding tissues.
7. Identify and preserve the infrahyoid muscles.
8. Excise the cyst along with a core of tissue surrounding the thyroglossal duct tract, extending from the cyst to the foramen cecum at the base of the tongue.
9. Remove the central portion of the hyoid bone (Sistrunk procedure) to ensure complete removal of the tract as seen in Fig. 1.14.
10. Ensure meticulous haemostasis to prevent post-operative haematoma formation.
11. Place a drain if necessary.
12. Close the wound in layers using absorbable sutures for deep tissue and non-absorbable sutures or staples for the skin.
13. Apply a sterile dressing.

Fig. 1.14 Thyroglossal duct cyst excised with the medial portion of hyoid bone. Illustrated by Vikum Liyanaarachchi

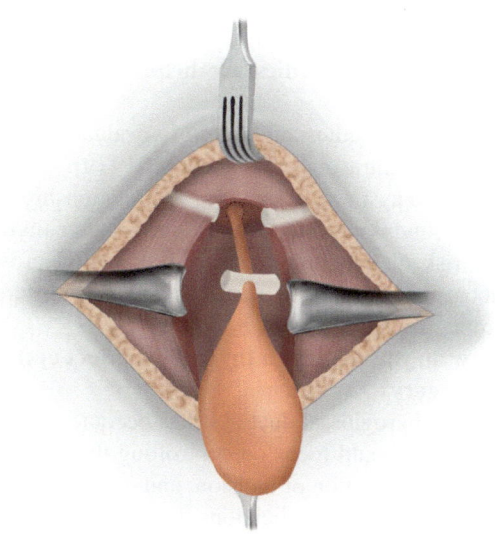

Important Points to Note During the Surgery

- Careful dissection and preservation of vital structures are crucial to avoid complications.
- Complete excision of the cyst and its tract, including the central portion of the hyoid bone, is essential to minimize the risk of recurrence.
- Meticulous haemostasis is important to prevent post-operative haematoma formation.

Questions a Consultant Might Ask a Trainee During the Operation

1. **Can you describe the embryological origin of the thyroglossal duct cyst?**
   The thyroglossal duct cyst is a congenital anomaly that results from the incomplete obliteration of the thyroglossal duct during embryonic development [19]. The thyroglossal duct is a temporary structure that forms during the descent of the thyroid gland from the foramen caecum at the base of the tongue to its final position in the neck. If the duct fails to involute completely, remnants can persist and form a cyst.
2. **What are the potential differential diagnoses for a midline neck mass, and how can they be differentiated preoperatively?**
   Potential differential diagnoses for a midline neck mass include dermoid cyst, lipoma, lymphadenopathy, sebaceous cyst, and enlarged thyroid nodule. A thorough history, physical examination, and imaging studies, such as ultrasound, computed tomography (CT), or magnetic resonance imaging (MRI), can help

differentiate these entities preoperatively. Fine-needle aspiration (FNA) biopsy may also be used for further evaluation.
3. **What imaging studies are helpful in evaluating a suspected thyroglossal duct cyst?**

   Imaging studies are helpful in evaluating a suspected thyroglossal duct cyst including ultrasound, CT, and MRI [19]. Ultrasound can provide information about the cyst's size, location, and relationship to adjacent structures. At least an ultrasound is needed to ensure that separate thyroid tissue is present to minimize the risk of hypothyroidism. CT and MRI provide more detailed information about the cyst and its tract and can help differentiate a thyroglossal duct cyst from other neck masses.
4. **How do you manage a thyroglossal duct cyst that has become infected prior to surgery?**

   If a thyroglossal duct cyst has become infected prior to surgery, initial management should focus on controlling the infection. This may involve antibiotic therapy, aspiration or incision, and drainage if an abscess has formed, and close monitoring for complications. Incision and drainage would ideally be avoided if possible as it would make the definitive excision surgery more challenging increasing the risk of recurrence. Once the infection has been adequately controlled, definitive surgical excision can be planned.
5. **What steps would you take if a pharyngeal or airway tear occurs during surgery?**
   - Preventive measures: Employ meticulous dissection techniques, especially on the deep aspect of the cyst, to minimize the risk of tears.
   - Primary closure: Attempt to close the tear primarily if the size and location permit.
   - Reinforcement: Use an overlying layer of strap muscle or a pedicled local flap such as one from the sternocleidomastoid (SCM) for additional reinforcement.
   - Tissue glue: Consider the application of tissue glue, such as Tisseel, to aid in sealing and healing the injury.
   - Drainage: Insert a non-suction corrugated drain to prevent fluid accumulation.
   - Post-operative care: Place a nasogastric (NG) tube, and perform a water-soluble swallow test post-operatively to assess for any ongoing issues or leaks if a pharyngeal injury is involved.
6. **Why is ultrasound important prior to thyroglossal duct cyst (TGDC) surgery?**

   Diagnostic confirmation: It helps confirm the diagnosis of TGDC and differentiates the cyst from other neck masses.

   Thyroid gland assessment: Ultrasound ensures that the thyroid gland is in situ and functioning. This is vital because if the TGDC is the only functioning thyroid tissue, removing it would necessitate lifelong thyroxine replacement. Patients must be informed about this potential outcome to make an informed decision about surgery.
7. **What are the anatomical variations of thyroglossal duct cysts (TGDCs)?**

TGDCs can vary in location relative to the hyoid bone:
- Infrahyoid: Present in 25–65% of cases, these are located below the hyoid bone.
- Suprahyoid: Found in 20–25% of cases, these cysts are located above the hyoid bone.
- At hyoid level: Approximately 15–20% of TGDCs are at the level of the hyoid bone itself.

8. **How can injury to the hypoglossal nerve be avoided during a Sistrunk procedure?**

    Meticulous dissection: Carefully dissect only the central portion of the hyoid bone. Avoid extending the dissection too far laterally beyond the lesser cornua of the hyoid bone, as this increases the risk of damaging the hypoglossal nerve. As the nerve courses down the neck, it passes close to the hyoid bone but typically lies superior and medial to it.

1.9 Lymph Node Biopsy

Indications for Surgery [20]

- Evaluation of unexplained lymphadenopathy
- Diagnosis of metastatic cancer or lymphoma
- Assessment of infectious or inflammatory conditions affecting the lymph nodes

Specific Risks Involved with the Surgery [20]

- Haemorrhage
- Infection
- Injury to adjacent structures (e.g. nerves, blood vessels)
- Seroma formation
- Scarring
- Chyle leak if low supraclavicular/level V lymphadenopathy

Steps of the Surgery

1. Administer local anaesthesia with or without sedation, or general anaesthesia, depending on the patient and the location of the lymph node.
2. Position the patient with a head ring and shoulder roll appropriately, depending on the location of the lymph node to be biopsied.
3. Consider injecting local anaesthetic such as Lignospan (1:80,000 adrenaline) or 1:100,000 adrenaline for haemostasis.
4. Identify the location of the target lymph node using palpation, ultrasound guidance, or preoperative imaging.
5. Make a small skin incision over the lymph node.

6. Dissect the subcutaneous tissue and fascia to expose the lymph node.
7. Carefully dissect around the lymph node, preserving the adjacent structures such as nerves and blood vessels.
8. Grasp the lymph node with forceps, and gently mobilize it from the surrounding tissue.
9. Excise the lymph node, and place it in a specimen container for pathological examination.
10. Achieve meticulous haemostasis to prevent post-operative haematoma formation.
11. Consider drain insertion if large dead space.
12. Close the wound in layers using absorbable sutures for deep tissue and non-absorbable sutures or staples for the skin.
13. Apply a sterile dressing.

Important Points to Note During the Surgery

- Careful dissection and preservation of vital structures are crucial to avoid complications.
- Meticulous haemostasis is important to prevent post-operative haematoma formation.
- Choose the most appropriate lymph node for biopsy to maximize diagnostic yield.

Questions a Consultant Might Ask a Trainee During the Operation

1. **What are the common causes of lymphadenopathy, and how can they be differentiated clinically?**
   Common causes of lymphadenopathy can be classified into three categories: infectious, inflammatory, and neoplastic. Infectious causes include bacterial, viral, fungal, or parasitic infections. Inflammatory causes include autoimmune or granulomatous diseases, such as lupus or sarcoidosis. Neoplastic causes include primary lymph node malignancies, such as lymphoma, or metastatic cancer from other primary sites. Clinical differentiation can be based on factors such as the location, size, and consistency of the lymph nodes, as well as the presence of systemic signs and symptoms.
2. **What are the different types of lymph node biopsies, and when is each type indicated?**
   There are different types of lymph node biopsies, including fine-needle aspiration biopsy (FNAB), core needle biopsy, and excisional or incisional biopsy. FNAB involves using a thin needle to aspirate cells from the lymph node, while core needle biopsy uses a larger needle to obtain a small tissue sample [20]. Excisional biopsy involves the removal of the entire lymph node, whereas incisional biopsy removes only a portion of the node. The choice of biopsy type

depends on factors such as the size and location of the lymph node, the clinical suspicion of the underlying pathology, and the need for a definitive diagnosis.

1.10 Transoral Robotic Surgery (TORS)

Indications for Surgery [21]

- Early-stage oropharyngeal cancer (e.g. tonsil, base of tongue)
- Attempting to identify a primary cancer in neck carcinoma of the unknown primary
- Obstructive sleep apnoea (OSA) unresponsive to conservative treatment
- Benign or malignant tumours of the pharynx or larynx
- Excision of certain parapharyngeal space tumours

Specific Risks Involved with the Surgery [21]

- Haemorrhage
- Infection
- Injury to adjacent structures (e.g. nerves, blood vessels, muscles, teeth, lips, and gums)
- Dysphagia (difficulty swallowing)
- Dysarthria (difficulty speaking)
- Dysgeusia (altered taste)
- Aspiration

Steps of the Surgery

1. Administer general anaesthesia, and perform endotracheal intubation.
2. Position the patient supine with the neck extended using a shoulder roll.
3. Insert a mouth gag, e.g. FK retractor, to provide adequate exposure of the oropharynx.
4. Dock the robotic surgical system, positioning the robotic arms and instruments to provide optimal access to the surgical site.
5. Excise the target lesion or perform the planned procedure (e.g. tumour resection, base of tongue reduction) using the robotic instruments under direct visualization.
6. Ensure complete removal of the lesion, and achieve adequate surgical margins, if applicable.
7. Perform meticulous haemostasis to prevent post-operative bleeding.
8. Close the surgical site, if necessary, using absorbable sutures.
9. Undock the robotic system, and remove the mouth gag.
10. Monitor the patient in the recovery room for any complications.

Important Points to Note During the Surgery

- Adequate exposure and visualization of the surgical site are crucial for a successful TORS procedure.
- Careful dissection and preservation of vital structures, such as nerves and blood vessels, are essential to minimize complications.
- Meticulous haemostasis is important to prevent post-operative bleeding.
- Proper patient selection and thorough preoperative planning are key to achieving good outcomes.

Questions a Consultant Might Ask a Trainee During the Operation

1. **What are the advantages of TORS compared to traditional open surgery or transoral laser microsurgery?**

    TORS has several advantages over traditional open surgery or transoral laser microsurgery. These advantages include improved visualization and access to the surgical site, enhanced precision and control due to the robotic system's ability to filter out hand tremors and scale movements, and reduced invasiveness, which can lead to faster recovery times, less pain, and decreased risk of complications. Additionally, TORS can be an organ-preserving approach, allowing patients to maintain better post-operative function and quality of life.

2. **What are the contraindications for TORS?**

    Contraindications for TORS include patients with significant medical comorbidities that preclude the safe administration of general anaesthesia, patients with large tumours that are not amenable to transoral resection, tumours involving critical structures that are not amenable to preservation, or patients with insufficient mouth opening or unfavourable anatomy that precludes the use of robotic instruments. Retropharyngeal internal carotid artery is an absolute contraindication to TORS lateral oropharyngectomy due to risk of catastrophic haemorrhage.

3. **Can you describe the role of TORS in the management of oropharyngeal cancer and its impact on post-operative function and quality of life?**

    TORS plays an important role in the management of oropharyngeal cancer, particularly in early-stage disease. It offers a minimally invasive approach for resecting tumours while preserving function and improving post-operative quality of life. By reducing the need for more extensive surgery, radiation, or chemoradiation, TORS can help patients maintain better speech and swallowing function, reduce the risk of long-term complications, and lead to faster recovery times.

1.11 Pharyngeal Pouch Surgery

1.11.1 Endoscopic Approach

Indications for Surgery [22]

- Dysphagia with associated weight loss
- Recurrent aspiration pneumonia
- Suspected malignancy
- Pouch size: at least one cervical vertebral body (>2.5 cm)

Specific Risks Involved with the Surgery [22]

- Failure of the procedure due to poor access
- Haemorrhage
- Infection
- Recurrence of symptoms
- Damage to teeth, lips, gums, and jaw/temporomandibular joint
- Oesophageal perforation

Steps of the Surgery

1. **Administer general anaesthesia**: Ensure that the patient is under general anaesthesia with appropriate monitoring.
2. **Position the patient**: Place the patient supine with a pillow beneath the shoulders to extend the neck. Use a mouth guard or wet swabs to protect the dentition.
3. **Perform rigid oesophagoscopy**: Identify the pouch, cricopharyngeal bar, and upper oesophagus, and rule out malignancy.
4. **Remove gastric contents**: Suction out any residual gastric contents from the pouch to prevent aspiration.
5. **Identify the pouch and oesophageal lumen**: Insert a nasogastric tube or anaesthetic bougie to delineate the anatomical structures.
6. **Insert diverticuloscope**: Place a Weerda diverticuloscope or Dohlman scope, and suspend it for optimal visualization.
7. **Apply endoscopic stapling device**: Position the stapling device across the cricopharyngeal bar, inverted, with the tip in the pharyngeal pouch.
8. **Assess the oesophageal mucosa**: Check for any breaches, and ensure adequate division and stapling of the cricopharyngeal bar. Perform additional stapling if necessary.
9. **Document with endoscopic photos**: Take pre- and post-stapling photographs for medical records.
10. **Check the oral structures**: Inspect the teeth, lips, gums, and jaw/temporomandibular joint for any damage.

11. **Post-operative care**: Keep the patient nil by mouth for a minimum of 2–4 h. Monitor for signs of oesophageal perforation, such as surgical emphysema.

1.11.2 Open Approach

Indications for Surgery

- Large (>4 cm or three cervical vertebral bodies) or recurrent pharyngeal pouch
- Poor intra-oral access
- Suspected malignancy

Specific Risks Involved with the Surgery

- Haemorrhage/haematoma
- Infection
- Recurrence of symptoms
- Scar
- Fistula
- Damage to teeth, lips, gums, and jaw/temporomandibular joint
- Oesophageal perforation
- Oesophageal stricture
- Recurrent laryngeal nerve palsy

Steps of the Surgery

1. **Administer general anaesthesia**: Ensure that the patient is under general anaesthesia with recurrent laryngeal nerve monitoring.
2. **Position the patient**: Place a pillow beneath the shoulders, and use a mouth guard or wet swabs to protect the dentition.
3. **Perform rigid oesophagoscopy**: Identify the pouch, cricopharyngeal bar, and upper oesophagus, and rule out malignancy.
4. **Remove gastric contents**: Suction out any residual gastric contents from the pouch.
5. **Pack the pouch**: Use ribbon gauze/BIPP and/or the rigid oesophagoscope to delineate the oesophageal lumen.
6. **Position for surgery**: Place a head ring and shoulder bolster with the head in a left lateral position.
7. **Inject local anaesthetic with adrenaline**: Mark the transverse incision site, and inject local anaesthetic with adrenaline for haemostasis.
8. **Make a transverse cervical incision**: Position the incision to the left of the midline at the level of the cricoid cartilage.

9. **Raise subplatysmal flaps**: Locate and divide the omohyoid muscle and middle thyroid vein. Identify the recurrent laryngeal nerve to facilitate rotation of the laryngotracheal complex and exposure of the pharyngeal pouch.
10. **Dissect and isolate the pouch**: Carefully dissect around the pouch to isolate it.
11. **Pouch management options**:
    (a) **Diverticulopexy**: Free and suspend the pouch.
    (b) **Diverticulectomy**: Invert the pouch into the oesophageal lumen and oversew, or resect using an endoscopic stapler or cold-steel excision with mattress suture closure.
12. **Perform cricopharyngeal myotomy**: Divide the muscle layer from below the cricopharyngeal muscle to the inferior border of the pouch neck.
13. **Close the neck incision**: Suture the incision in layers, and insert a neck drain.
14. **Insert a nasogastric tube**: For post-operative feeding and decompression.
15. **Post-operative care**: Keep the patient nil by mouth with nasogastric feeding for 5–7 days. Monitor for oesophageal perforation, and perform a water-soluble swallow test.

Important Points to Note During Surgery

- **Proper visualization**: Ensure optimal positioning and suspension of the diverticuloscope for clear visualization of the surgical field.
- **Use of intraoperative imaging**: Endoscopic photos pre- and post-stapling help in documenting the procedure and verifying the results.
- **Post-operative monitoring**: Careful observation for signs of oesophageal perforation and other complications is essential for early detection and management.

Questions a Consultant Might Ask a Trainee During the Operation

1. **What are the signs and symptoms of a pharyngeal pouch, and how is the diagnosis confirmed?**
    A patient with a pharyngeal pouch commonly presents with regurgitation and halitosis due to food accumulation in the pouch [22]. Progressive dysphagia and choking worsen as the pouch enlarges. Chronic aspiration of pouch contents can lead to a chronic cough and recurrent aspiration pneumonia. Other symptoms include weight loss, neck swelling (large pouch), and gurgling sounds in the neck (Boyce's sign). Diagnosis is confirmed with a fluoroscopic swallow test using barium.
2. **What is the pathophysiology of a pharyngeal pouch?**
    A pharyngeal pouch forms as a pulsion diverticulum through a natural weakness in the pharyngeal mucosa between the cricopharyngeus and thyropharyngeus muscles (Killian's dehiscence), both part of the inferior constrictor of the pharynx [22].
3. **How do you size a pharyngeal pouch, and why is this relevant?**

Pharyngeal pouch size is classified using systems such as the Van Overbeek classification, which compares pouch length to cervical vertebrae on X-ray, with small pouches being shorter than one vertebra and large pouches being longer than three vertebrae. The Morton-Bartney classification divides pouches into small (<2.5 cm), medium (2.5–4 cm), and large (>4 cm). Pouch size is relevant as small pouches (<2.5 cm) may not accommodate an endoscopic stapler, necessitating other approaches like CO2 laser or an open procedure. Large pouches may require an open approach.

4. **What are the signs of oesophageal perforation, and how is it managed?**

   Early signs of oesophageal perforation include tachycardia, tachypnoea, and fever. Patients may experience retrosternal chest pain or chest pain radiating to the back, along with surgical emphysema in the neck (feeling like bubble wrap).

   Management involves:
   - Keeping the patient nil by mouth.
   - Placing a nasogastric tube or using total parenteral nutrition via a central line.
   - Administering prophylactic antibiotics.
   - Performing an urgent water-soluble (Gastrografin) swallow test.
   - Significant perforations may require open surgical repair with multidisciplinary involvement (upper GI surgery or thoracic surgery).
   - Smaller perforations can be managed conservatively with antibiotics, nil by mouth, and observation with serial imaging.
   - An unrecognised oesophageal perforation can lead to mediastinitis and potentially death.

5. **What are the alternative management options for a pharyngeal pouch?**

   Alternative management options include:
   - **Small pouches (<2.5 cm)**: CO2 laser treatment.
   - **Recurrent or large pouches, or difficult oral access**: Open approach.
   - **Conservative management**: For elderly patients with significant comorbidities contraindicating general anaesthesia, managed by speech and language therapists who guide food and fluid consistency and advice strategies to minimize aspiration.

6. **What are the different types of pharyngeal pouches, and how are they created?**

   Pharyngeal pouches can be classified based on their anatomical location and formation mechanism:
   - **Zenker's diverticulum**: The most common type occurs above the cricopharyngeus muscle through Killian's dehiscence, a natural weakness between the fibres of the cricopharyngeus and thyropharyngeus muscles.
   - **Killian-Jamieson diverticulum**: Less common, occurs below the cricopharyngeus muscle and through Killian-Jamieson area, a natural gap between the cricopharyngeus and the cervical oesophagus.
   - **Laimer's diverticulum**: Very rare, occurs below the cricopharyngeus muscle and through Laimer's triangle, an area bordered by the longitudinal muscles of the oesophagus.

References

1. Li LQ, Hilmi O, England J, Tolley N. An update on the management of thyroid nodules: rationalising the guidelines. J Laryngol Otol. 2023;137(9):965–70.
2. Arrangoiz R, Cordera F, Caba D, Muñoz M, Moreno E, de León EL. Comprehensive review of thyroid embryology, anatomy, histology, and physiology for surgeons. Int J Otolaryngol Head Neck Surg. 2018;7(4):160–88.
3. Taterra D, Wong LM, Vikse J, et al. The prevalence and anatomy of parathyroid glands: a meta-analysis with implications for parathyroid surgery. Langenbeck's Arch Surg. 2019;404:63–70.
4. Randolph GW. Surgery of the thyroid and parathyroid glands. Elsevier Health Sciences; 2020.
5. National Institute for Health and Care Excellence (NICE). Hyperparathyroidism (primary): diagnosis, assessment and initial management. NICE guideline [NG132]. 2019 May. Available from: https://www.nice.org.uk/guidance/ng132
6. British Association of Endocrine and Thyroid Surgeons (BAETS). Guidelines for the management of postoperative hypocalcaemia. BAETS guideline. 2017. Available from: https://www.baets.org.uk/guidelines/hypocalcaemia-management
7. Ferlito A, Rinaldo A, Robbins KT, Silver CE. Neck dissection: past, present and future? J Laryngol Otol. 2006;120(2):87–92.
8. Krmpotic-Nemanic J, Draf W, Helms J. Surgical anatomy of head and neck. Springer Science & Business Media; 2012.
9. Amin MB, Edge SB, Greene FL, et al., editors. AJCC cancer staging manual. 8th ed. New York: Springer; 2017.
10. Beahm DD, Peleaz L, Nuss DW, et al. Surgical approaches to the submandibular gland: a review of literature. Int J Surg. 2009;7(6):503–9.
11. Grewal JS, Jamal Z, Ryan J. Anatomy, head and neck, submandibular gland. In: StatPearls. Treasure Island (FL): StatPearls Publishing; 2023.
12. Cracchiolo JR, Shaha AR. Parotidectomy for parotid cancer. Otolaryngol Clin N Am. 2016;49(2):415–24.
13. Kochhar A, Larian B, Azizzadeh B. Facial nerve and parotid gland anatomy. Otolaryngol Clin N Am. 2016;49(2):273–84.
14. Palmer TJ, Pathak KA, Sood S, et al. Management of salivary gland tumours: United Kingdom national multidisciplinary guidelines. J Laryngol Otol. 2016;130(S2):S142–9.
15. Available from: https://www.cambridge.org/core/journals/journal-of-laryngology-and-otology/head-and-neck-guidelines
16. Mohebati A, Shah JP. Total laryngectomy. Int J Otorhinolaryngol Clin. 2011;2(3):207–14.
17. Zaifullah S, Yunus MR, See GB. Diagnosis and treatment of branchial cleft anomalies in UKMMC: a 10-year retrospective study. Eur Arch Otorrinolaringol. 2013;270:1501–6.
18. Bagchi A, Hira P, Mittal K, Priyamvara A, Dey AK. Branchial cleft cysts: a pictorial review. Pol J Radiol. 2018;83:e204–9.
19. Goldsztein H, Khan A, Pereira KD. Thyroglossal duct cyst excision—the Sistrunk procedure. Oper Tech Otolaryngol Head Neck Surg. 2009;20(4):256–9.
20. Pitman KT, Ferlito A, Devaney KO, Shaha AR, Rinaldo A. Sentinel lymph node biopsy in head and neck cancer. Oral Oncol. 2003;39(4):343–9.
21. Yee S. Transoral robotic surgery. AORN J. 2017;105(1):73–84.
22. Aly A, Devitt PG, Jamieson GG. Evolution of surgical treatment for pharyngeal pouch. J Br Surg. 2004;91(6):657–64.

Otology 2

Iain Mckay-Davies, Zohaib Siddiqui, Basim Wahba, and Keli Dusu

2.1 Myringotomy and Tube Placement

Indications for Surgery [1, 2]

- Middle ear effusion causing hearing loss affecting speech and language development in children
- Recurrent acute otitis media (RAOM) (3 AOM episodes in the last 6 months or at least 4 AOM episodes in the last 12 months with at least 1 in the last 6 months)
- Complicated AOM, including mastoiditis, or sigmoid thrombosis, and meningitis (often combined with cortical mastoidectomy)
- Chronic otitis media with effusion (OME) not responsive to conservative treatment
- Barotrauma in patients with Eustachian tube dysfunction
- Retracted tympanic membrane
- Meniere's—pressure relief and steroid injection delivery

Specific Risks Involved with the Surgery [1]

- Bleeding
- Infection
- Recurrence of effusions
- Persistent tympanic membrane perforation
- Myringosclerotic patches
- Cholesteatoma formation: rare

Steps of the Surgery

1. Administration of local [topical EMLA cream to tympanic membrane, xylocaine/lignospan local anaesthetic injection to posterior canal] or general anaesthesia.
2. Patient positioning: supine with the head turned to one side using head ring.
3. Insertion of largest speculum possible into the ear canal or endoscopic approach.
4. Inspect attic region and pars tensa for retractions, cholesteatoma/perforation/ other abnormalities.
5. Myringotomy incision with myringotome, classically at the anteroinferior quadrant of the tympanic membrane. A vertical incision at the 6 o'clock position can also be used. It is a common practice as well to do the myringotomy posteriorly (for easier repair if persistent perforation occurs). Keep in mind if posterior to avoid injury to the ossicular chain (posterior superior quadrant).
6. Using fine-tip suction, aspirate fluid from the middle if present.
7. Insertion of the tympanostomy/ventilation tube (as seen in Fig. 2.1).
8. Reassessment of tympanic membrane and tube placement.
9. Insertion of non-ototoxic antibiotic drops or saline (reduces obstruction).
10. Repeat steps 3–9 on the contralateral side, if bilateral procedure.

Important Points to Note During the Surgery

- Avoid incising the handle of the malleus or the round window niche.
- Ensure correct placement and orientation of the tube.
- Minimize handling of the tympanic membrane to prevent scarring and ensure that the myringotomy is not too wide (else risks early extrusion).

Questions a Consultant Might Ask a Trainee About the Operation

1. **Why is the anteroinferior quadrant chosen for the myringotomy incision?**
   This location minimizes the risk of injury to important structures, such as the ossicles, facial nerve, and round window niche; however, inferior or postero-

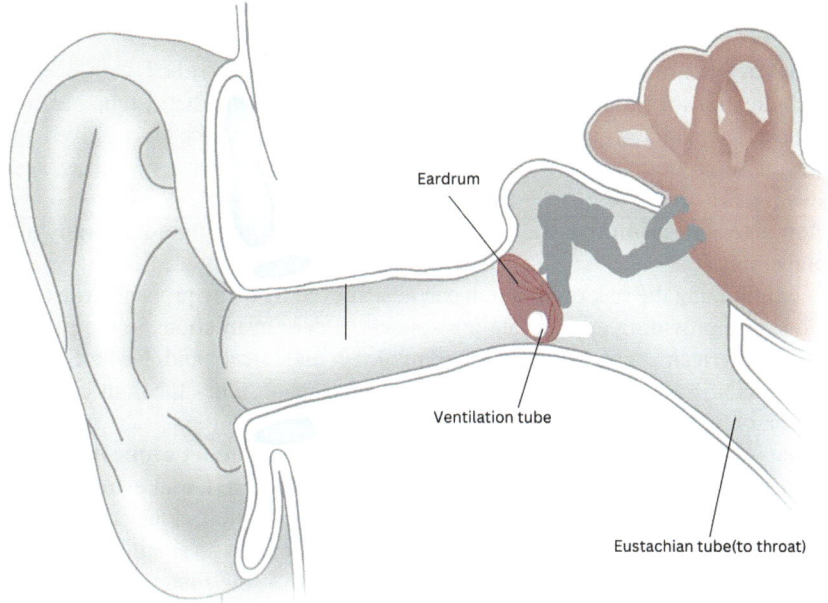

Fig. 2.1 Ventilation tube in situ in tympanic membrane. Illustrated by Vikum Liyanaarachchi

Fig. 2.2 Examples of different grommets used: Shah grommet, titanium grommet, T-tube (left to right). Illustrated by Vikum Liyanaarachchi

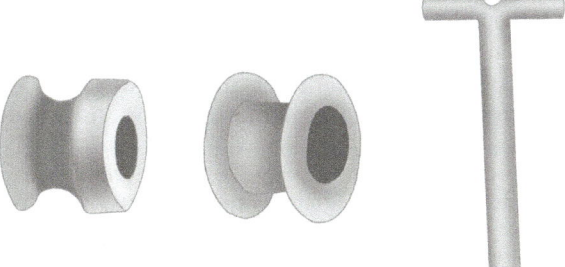

inferior is also a common site preferred by many authors as it is easier to repair inferior/posterior perforation than anterior one if it does not heal by itself.

2. **What are the common types of tympanostomy tubes?**

    The common types include Shah, mini-Shah, Shea, Shepard, Collar Button, and T-tubes and Triunes, each with varying shapes and sizes designed for specific indications and patient populations. Common examples can be seen in Fig. 2.2.

3. **How long do tympanostomy tubes typically remain in place?**

Tubes generally remain in place for 9–12 months, depending on the type of tube and individual patient factors. T-tubes and Triunes are designed to stay longer [1].

4. **What are the indications for removing a tympanostomy tube?**

   Indications for removal include persistent/recurrent otorrhoea, tube obstruction, and someone whose initial indication for ventilation tube has resolved and they now request a dry waterproof ear that they can swim with (i.e. keen swimmers).

5. **How can you minimize the risk of infection after myringotomy and tube placement?**

   Minimizing the risk of infection can be achieved by using proper sterile technique and providing appropriate post-operative care instructions to the patient. [See American Academy of Otolaryngology and Head and Neck Surgery (AA-OHNS) clinical practice guidelines for tympanostomy tubes in children, February 2022.]

6. **What is the role of adenoidectomy in children with Grommet's tube insertion?**

   According to NICE guidelines 2023 [based on TARGET trial evidence], the duration of benefit of grommets persists even after extrusion, if the adenoids are removed at the same time. The benefit of adenoidectomy is so significant that the NICE guidelines 2023 recommend adenoidectomy at the first set of grommet insertion [2]. When planning grommets for the management of OME, consider adjuvant adenoidectomy unless assessment indicates an abnormality with the palate.

   According to AA-OHNS guidelines 2022 [3], clinician needs to perform adenoidectomy as an adjunct to tympanostomy tube insertion for children with symptoms directly related to the adenoid (adenoid infection or nasal obstruction) or in children aged 4 years or older to reduce future incidence of recurrent otitis media or the need for repeat tube insertion.

7. **What is the first line of management otitis media with effusion in children with Down's syndrome?**

   Hearing aid is to be offered as the first line of management in children with Down's syndromes. [NICE] Grommet tube insertion is relatively challenging due to narrow external ear (mini-Shah grommets to be considered). There is also higher incidence of early grommet tube extrusion, higher recurrence rate of glue ear (due to chronic Eustachian tube dysfunction due to generalized hypotonia), and higher incidence of infection and otorrhoea (due to reduced immunity).

2.2 Tympanoplasty (Types I, II, III, IV, V)

It is worth noting that the different types of tympanoplasty can be discussed in your exams (Table 2.1). However, the term is not commonly used in practice.

Indications for Surgery [3]

- Chronic tympanic membrane perforation

Table 2.1 Tympanoplasty classification based on Wullstein 1956 and revised by Mirko Toss, MD [3]. Figure 2.3 illustrates the reconstruction

Type	Tympanoplasty
Type I *Myringoplasty*	Tympanic membrane (TM) repair only—Intact ossicular chain
Type II *Myringo-incudopexy*	Ossicular chain repair of the lever mechanism. Malleus partially eroded. TM +/− malleus remnant grafted to incus
Type III (minor columella) *Myringo-stapediopexy*	Ossicular chain repair performed by placing a graft from stapes capitulum to TM or manubrium
Type III (major columella)	Ossicular chain repair performed by placing a graft between stapes footplate and TM or manubrium
Type III (stapes columella)	Ossicular chain repair performed by placing a graft onto the capitulum of the stapes
Type IV	Graft placed onto round window. Stapes footplate is mobile
Type Va *Fenestration*	Stapes footplate is fixed and has no ossicles; a fenestration of the stapes footplate (stapedotomy) or lateral semicircular canal is performed
Type Vb	There is a fixed footplate which is removed. This has replaced type Va. The round window is covered with a graft

- Conductive hearing loss due to ossicular chain disruption or perforation
- Cholesteatoma or chronic otitis media
- Retraction pocket

Specific Risks Involved with the Surgery [3]

- Bleeding
- Infection
- Scar
- Pain
- Pinna numbness
- Hearing loss
- Tinnitus
- Vertigo or dizziness
- Facial nerve injury: rare
- Graft failure
- Temporary altered taste
- Need for regular microsuction
- Recurrence
- Need for second-look surgery/DWI MRI
- Taste disturbance (chorda-tympani injury)

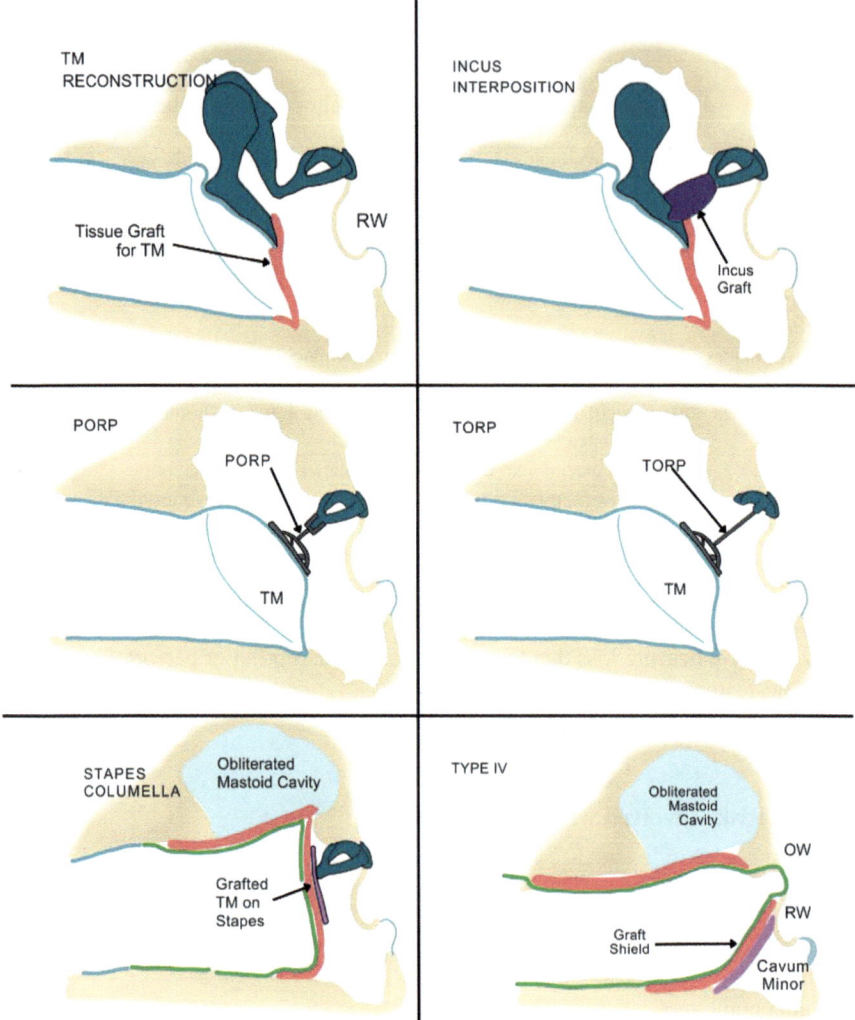

Fig. 2.3 Different types of tympanoplasty reconstruction. Illustrated by Vikum Liyanaarachchi

2.2.1 Preoperative Preparation

- **Hearing tests**: Perform audiometric tests to assess the extent of hearing loss and to ensure that this is not the only hearing ear.
- **Anaesthesia**: Administer local or hypotensive general anaesthesia, based on patient and surgeon preference.
- **Patient positioning**: Place the patient supine with the head turned to one side and supported by a head ring to provide optimal surgical access.

Surgical Steps

1. **Selection of surgical approach:** Choose between endaural, postauricular, or permeatal approaches based on the location and size of the perforation and surgeon's preference (Figs. 2.4 and 2.5).
2. If posterior auricular incision is used, you will need to perform a re-entry incision into the ear canal.
3. **Tympanomeatal flap elevation**: Carefully elevate the tympanomeatal flap up to the annulus to expose the middle ear space as seen in Fig. 2.6.
4. **Middle ear exploration**: Explore the middle ear and ossicular chain for any pathologies or ossicular discontinuity. Be careful with regard to the chorda-tympani as it can be easily damaged.
5. **Perforation edge freshening**: Use a fine needle or pick to carefully freshen the edges of the TM perforation to promote graft adherence and healing.
6. **Graft Preparation and Placement**
   - **Graft selection:** Choose a graft material, commonly temporalis fascia, cartilage, or perichondrium. Each has its advantages in terms of availability, ease of harvest, and post-operative outcomes.
   - **Temporalis fascia graft:** Most commonly used due to its ease of harvest and good integration. Harvested from the temporalis muscle fascia through a small incision above the ear or using the initial postauricular incision.

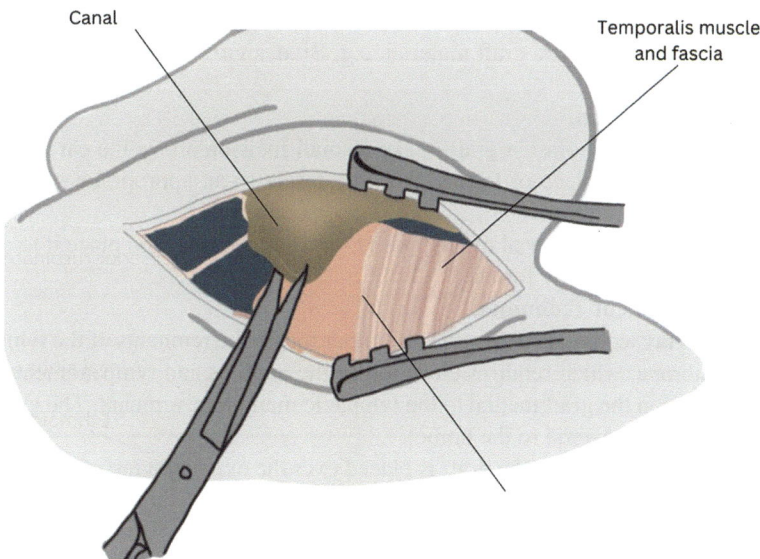

Fig. 2.4 View of posterior auricular incision, temporalis muscle visible superiorly, and canal wall. Re-entry incision made through canal wall. Illustrated by Vikum Liyanaarachchi

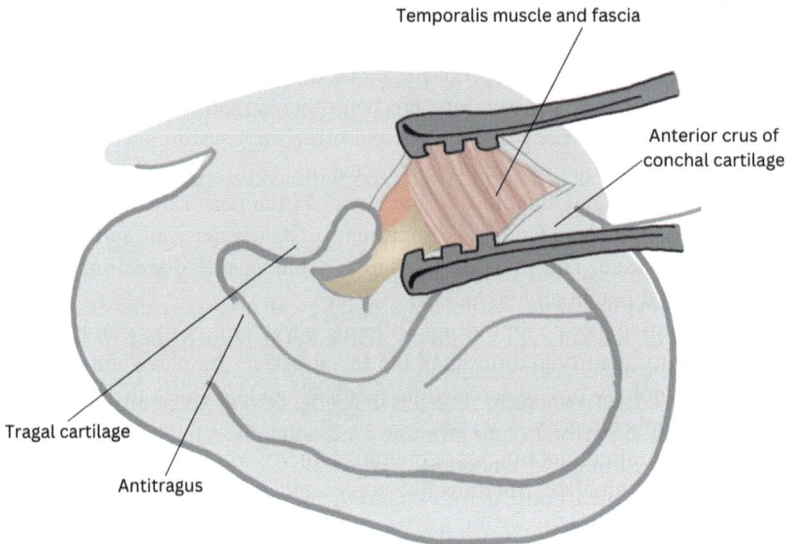

Fig. 2.5 End-aural incision. Illustrated by Vikum Liyanaarachchi

- **Cartilage graft:** Offers increased rigidity and resistance to retraction or resorption. Typically harvested from the tragus or conchal bowl. Often used in revision cases.
- **Perichondrium graft:** A thin layer of tissue covering cartilage, used for its pliability and ability to conform to irregular perforations. Sourced from the tragus.
- **Allograft:** Synthetic graft material, e.g. Biodesign™ (porcine-derived extracellular matrix).

7. **Graft Preparation:**
   - For a temporalis fascia graft, make a small incision above the ear to expose and harvest a piece of fascia. Trim the fascia to an appropriate size, larger than the perforation.
   - Clean the graft material of any muscle or fibrous tissue, and place it to dry or in saline until ready for use.
8. **Graft Placement Techniques:**
   - **Underlay** technique: Place the graft underneath the remnants of the tympanic membrane, which requires elevation of the annulus and tympanomeatal flap to position the graft medial to the tympanic membrane remnant. The graft can be medial or lateral to the umbo.
   - **Overlay** technique: The graft is placed over the existing tympanic membrane remnants and the annular ring. This technique is less commonly used due to a higher risk of lateralization of the graft.
   - **Inlay technique**: Used for small perforations where the graft is placed directly into the perforation, described as a butterfly inlay graft. The surgeon

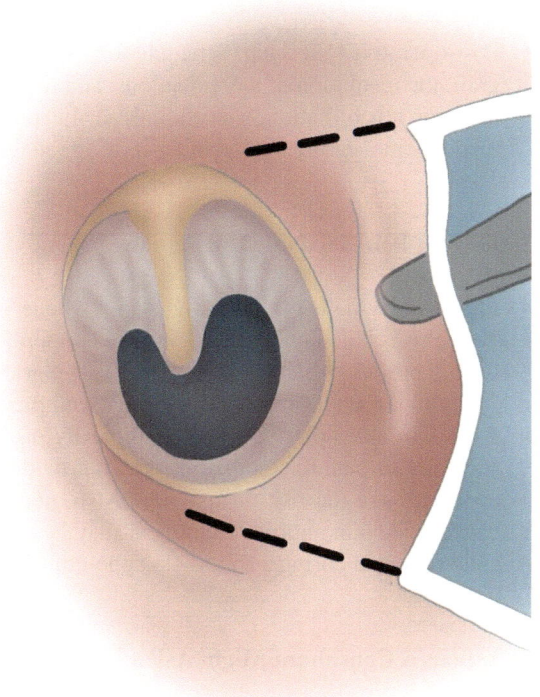

Fig. 2.6 Creation of a tympanomeatal flap being raised towards the annulus. Illustrated by Vikum Liyanaarachchi

would insert the cartilage graft into the perforation edges of TM by creating circumferential grooves on the cartilage graft.
- Graft stabilization: Secure the graft in place using gel foam or a similar absorbable material to support the graft during the healing process.

2.2.2 Post-Operative Steps

1. Tympanomeatal flap repositioning and closure: Carefully reposition the tympanomeatal flap over the graft, and secure it in place.
2. Packing: Place absorbable or non-absorbable packing material in the ear canal to support the flap and graft and to absorb any discharge.
3. Post-operative care instructions: Provide the patient with instructions regarding activity restrictions, ear protection, and follow-up appointments for graft and hearing evaluation. No flying or swimming for 2 months post-op.

Follow-Up and Rehabilitation

- Post-operative follow-up: Schedule follow-up visits to monitor the healing of the graft, the resolution of any infections, and the restoration of hearing.
- Hearing rehabilitation: Depending on the post-operative hearing assessment, recommend hearing aids or other hearing rehabilitation services if necessary.

Important Points to Note During the Surgery

- Preserve the malleus handle and stapes whenever possible.
- The graft is commonly taken from the temporal fascia/tragal cartilage.
- Ensure proper sizing and positioning of the graft and prosthesis.
- Injury to the stapes footplate can cause complete deafness.
- After a tympanoplasty, the ear is typically packed with an absorbable material such as Gelfoam to stabilize the graft, provide support for the healing process, and minimize the risk of infection. Also, non-absorbable materials like ribbon gauze soaked in antibiotic ointment may be used. The packing material is typically removed during a follow-up appointment a few weeks after surgery.

Questions a Consultant Might Ask a Trainee About the Operation

1. **What are the common materials used for the graft in tympanoplasty?**
   Common graft materials include temporalis fascia, tragal perichondrium, cymbal or tragal cartilage, and synthetic materials such as bioengineered tissue.
2. **How do you determine the type of tympanoplasty needed for a patient?**
   The type of tympanoplasty is determined by the extent of the tympanic membrane perforation, ossicular chain involvement, and presence/extent of cholesteatoma or other middle ear pathology.
3. **How do you choose between the different approaches: postauricular (PA), endaural (EA), and permeatal (PM)?**
   The postauricular (PA) approach is preferred for extensive diseases like large cholesteatomas or chronic otitis media needing comprehensive middle ear or mastoid surgery. It offers excellent exposure but is more invasive, leading to a longer recovery and visible scarring behind the ear. It will also be required if the ear canal is narrow.
   The endaural (EA) approach suits surgeries primarily on the posterior or central parts of the tympanic membrane or ossicular chain reconstruction. It provides good exposure with a cosmetically appealing incision inside the ear canal and extending to the helical root, leading to a potentially quicker recovery. However, it may not offer sufficient exposure for extensive anterior diseases. The only advantage of the EA approach over the PM approach is that instead of operating through a speculum which requires a finger/mechanical arm to hold it, a retractor can be inserted into the wound. The access is no greater.

The permeatal (PM) approach is a minimally invasive tympanoplasty technique performed through the ear canal. It is best for small tympanic membrane perforations or limited middle ear issues, offering a quick recovery and minimal discomfort without external scarring. This approach is limited to cases where extensive visibility and access to the ear structures are not required. All approaches can be combined with endoscopic techniques.

4. **How do you manage a patient with persistent conductive hearing loss after tympanoplasty?**

    Patients with persistent conductive hearing loss may benefit from revision surgery, hearing aids, or bone conduction devices.

5. **What is the role of preoperative imaging in tympanoplasty?**

    Preoperative imaging, such as computed tomography (CT), can help assess the extent of middle ear pathology, ossicular chain involvement, and plan the surgical approach. It is important for key structures to be visualized such as the facial nerve—is there any dehiscence? Up to 40% of the population can have bony dehiscence of the facial canal. The position of the sigmoid sinus and the dura is also important to consider. The position of the tegmen tympani and if there is a lateral semicircular canal fistula can also be evaluated on a CT. However, CT is not required for myringoplasty, but it is for anything other than a simple perforation.

6. **What is the age you recommend performing tympanoplasty in a child with persistent perforation following grommet tube extrusion?**

    The decision and chances of success of the surgery depend on the status of the other ear and Eustachian tube function. We must consider the patient's quality of life, e.g. hearing impairment and keen swimmer.

    Many would offer the surgery to a patient from the age of 5 years or older. Ninety-three percent of perforations will heal within 2 years; if it has not healed by this time, then offering a surgical option is possible. Leaving a child with a chronic discharging ear, avoiding water/swimming, and potentially worse hearing for many years arguably are not wise. It can be technically challenging to perform this operation on children younger than this.

7. **What surgical options are available in cases of anterior or large tympanic membrane perforation?**

    By performing anterosuperior tunnelled pull-through (Kerr) flap if the perforation is anterior or complete cuff (circumferential tunnel) and if the perforation is large/subtotal to support the graft circumferentially on the ear canal.

8. **What is the difference in the posterior auricular incision when performed in children for myringoplasty?**

    The incision is the same. However, if performing mastoidectomy or cochlear implantation in children <2 years old, then the incision is done more superiorly and does not extend inferiorly as the mastoid tip is still underdeveloped leaving the facial nerve more lateral and superficial and thus prone to injury.

2.3 Mastoidectomy

Indications for Surgery [4]

- Cholesteatoma/active squamous chronic otitis media (COM)
  - **Active mucosal COM**: Persistent ear discharge (otorrhoea), Inflammation, and infection are ongoing.
  - **Inactive mucosal COM**: Dry perforation without active discharge. Minimal symptoms.
  - **Active squamous COM (i.e. cholesteatoma)**:
    (a) **Cholesteatoma** is an abnormal growth of squamous epithelium within the middle ear or mastoid cavity.
    (b) It can be **active** (with ongoing inflammation and discharge) or **inactive/stable** (retraction pocket).
- Acute mastoiditis
- Complications of middle ear infection (e.g. facial nerve palsy, intracranial involvement, acute mastoiditis, sigmoid sinus thrombosis, AOM with mastoiditis failing to resolve with medical management)
- Access for cochlear implantation or other middle/inner ear/mastoid surgeries
- Temporal bone resection surgery
- Finding the facial nerve

Specific Risks Involved with the Surgery [4]

- Bleeding
- Infection
- Scar, pain, pinna numbness
- Hearing loss
- Tinnitus
- Vertigo or dizziness
- Facial nerve injury
- Taste disturbance (chorda tympani injury)
- Cerebrospinal fluid (CSF) leak (due to damage to tegmen and underlying dura)
- Residual/recurrent disease

Diamond Drill Usage in Mastoidectomy

- The diamond drill is employed for its precision and safety, particularly near critical structures like the facial nerve and the dura.
- It generates less heat, reducing the risk of thermal injury to inner ear structures.
- Ideal for finer bone work and smoothing bone surfaces after initial drilling with a cutting burr.
- Essential in delicate areas and for final touches, ensuring minimal trauma to the surrounding tissues.

Canal Wall-Up (CWU) Mastoidectomy

- Preserves the posterior ear canal wall.
- Indicated for limited cholesteatoma cases/small retraction pockets.

Canal Wall-Down (CWD) Mastoidectomy

- Removes the posterior ear canal wall for extensive disease.
- Used in extensive cholesteatoma or high-risk intracranial complications.

Common Surgical Steps

1. Hypotensive GA administration
2. Patient positioning for optimal access on head ring with head turned away
3. Postauricular incision
4. Mastoid cortex exposure
5. Initial drilling with a cutting burr (5–6 mm), followed by precision work with a diamond drill and identification of critical landmarks (middle fossa dura, sigmoid sinus, facial nerve, lateral canal). The drilling is focused in Macewen's Triangle, bounded by the posterior root of the zygoma (suprameatal spine), the posterior wall of the external auditory canal, and a line tangential to the canal's posterior edge, providing safe access to the mastoid antrum. Carefully identify key landmarks, including the middle fossa dura, sigmoid sinus, facial nerve, and lateral semicircular canal, to ensure anatomical preservation.

Procedure-Specific Steps

- CWU: If possible, conserving middle ear structures, removing pathological tissues, surgical closure
- CWD: Extensive drilling, creating a unified cavity, surgical closure

Critical Surgical Considerations

- Complete pathological tissue removal to prevent leaving residual disease.
- Choice between CWU and CWD based on the disease extent and chances of complete removal. A CWU for small, well-defined disease. If extensive, friable disease and previous failed CWU operations, then a CWD.
- Preserve the facial nerve and other critical structures (e.g. dura, sigmoid sinus, stapes, lateral canal).
- Minimize handling of the middle ear structures to prevent scarring and adhesions.
- Ensure complete removal of the cholesteatoma or infected tissue to prevent recurrence or leaving residual disease.

Questions a Consultant Might Ask a Trainee About the Operation

1. **What are the main differences between canal wall-up (CWU) and canal wall-down (CWD) mastoidectomy, and how is the appropriate technique determined?**

    In a canal wall-up (CWU) mastoidectomy, the focus is on removing air cells in the mastoid while preserving the posterior canal wall. This technique also aims to retain the tympanic membrane and, where possible, the ossicular chain. It is typically indicated for children, keen swimmers, first surgery for a newly diagnosed cholesteatoma, and limited/clearly defined cholesteatoma [4].

    Conversely, the canal wall-down (CWD) mastoidectomy involves a comprehensive removal of mastoid air cells and the posterior canal wall. This procedure results in an enlarged cavity that merges with the external ear canal. It is preferred in extensive cholesteatoma cases; in cases with a sclerotic, small mastoid and low tegmen (rendering a CWU approach technically difficult); for failed CWU procedures with extensive residual disease; or if the patient's comorbidities or patient's wishes necessitate one comprehensive surgery.

2. **During mastoidectomy, how can you minimize the risk of injury to the facial nerve and other critical structures?**

    To minimize the risk of injury, first identify the key anatomical landmarks, such as the sigmoid sinus, posterior canal wall, and lateral semicircular canal [5]. Use a 4 mm diamond burr for drilling vertically (parallel to the underlying facial nerve) behind the posterior canal wall, below the inferior edge of the lateral SCC, and employ gentle and controlled movements. Constantly irrigate the area to reduce the risk of thermal injury. Watch for the nerve (light pink) or the tiny vessels that lie within its sheath. Monitoring the facial nerve function intraoperatively and using a facial nerve stimulator set to 0.5 mA can also be helpful.

3. **What are the potential consequences of leaving residual cholesteatoma after mastoidectomy, and how do you manage it?**

    Residual cholesteatoma can lead to recurrence of the symptoms, persistent infection, hearing loss, and potentially life-threatening complications such as intracranial spread. If residual cholesteatoma is suspected or confirmed, revision surgery may be necessary to remove the remaining cholesteatoma and prevent further complications.

4. **What are some factors that may contribute to surgical failure or complications following mastoidectomy?**

    Factors that may contribute to surgical failure or complications include incomplete removal of the cholesteatoma or infected tissue, Eustachian tube dysfunction, and poor patient compliance with post-operative care instructions, leading to wound infections.

5. **How do you manage a patient with persistent conductive hearing loss after a mastoidectomy?**

    For patients with persistent conductive hearing loss after mastoidectomy, the following options can be considered [6]:
    - Revision surgery to address ossicular chain issues or residual disease
    - Hearing aids to amplify sound

- Bone conduction devices to bypass the conductive hearing loss and directly stimulate the cochlea

    The choice of management depends on the patient's preferences, the degree of hearing loss, and the cause of the hearing loss.

6. **What are the anatomical landmarks of the facial nerve?**
    - Posterosuperior to processus cochleariformis
    - Superior to oval window
    - Inferior to the lateral semicircular canal
    - Immediately medial to the digastric ridge [5]

7. **What are the landmarks for posterior tympanotomy?**
    - Facial nerve medially
    - Chorda tympani laterally
    - Fossa incudis and short process of the incus superiorly

    A posterior tympanotomy allows access to the mesotympanum.

8. **What is the subiculum and ponticulus?**

    These landmarks are better visualized during endoscopic ear surgery. The subiculum is a ridge which separates between round window and styloid eminence. It lies inferior to the sinus tympani. Ponticulus is a ridge between the pyramidal process and the oval window. It lies superior to the sinus tympani. Sinus tympani are a common site for residual cholesteatoma.

9. **What do you do if you encounter a CSF leak?**

    With any complication in surgery, the first step is to inform the team and anaesthetist.

    Investigate the injury, and inspect the dura. Ultimately, you will want to place a multi-layered covering/graft over the defect. This can be done in different ways. We would suggest fascia inlay, bone pâté, and then fascia to overlay, with Tisseel glue at each step.

    If small, can plug with free temporalis muscle graft, and glue in place with Tisseel.

10. **What are the most common sites for residual cholesteatoma?**

    Sinus tympani, facial recess, anterior epitympanic recess, peri Eustachian tube, hypotympanum, digastric ridge

11. **What is the cog and its clinical significance?**

    In mastoidectomy, particularly in the canal wall-up (CWU) approach, the "cog" refers to a sheet of bone that lies anterior to the head of the malleus and hangs from the tegmen. It separates the anterior attic (anterior epitympanic space) from the posterior attic (posterior epitympanic space). It points down towards the cochleariform process, and cholesteatoma can be hidden behind it.

12. **What is the isthmus and tensor fold and their clinical significance?**

    In the context of mastoid surgery, the isthmus is the narrow passage connecting the tympanic cavity to the mastoid air cells, critical for ventilation. It is a mucosal fold that lies between the incus and malleus, and if complete, it can impede the ventilation pathways from the middle ear to attic, thus contributing to attic retraction pocket formation. The tensor fold is a mucosal fold around the tensor tympani muscle, which if complete impedes ventilation from the middle ear/Eustachian tube to the attic, contributing to retraction pocket formation. Clinically, ensuring that these structures are opened during surgery is vital for maintaining proper attic ventilation and preventing retraction pocket recurrence.

13. **What is the path of the chorda tympani?**

    During mastoidectomy or tympanoplasty, it is crucial to avoid damaging the chorda tympani (CT) to prevent the loss of taste sensation on the anterior two-thirds of the tongue or decreased salivation.

    Anatomical pathway of the CT:
    - The CT enters the middle ear through the petrotympanic fissure.
    - It then passes underneath the neck of the malleus and over the long process of the incus.
    - The CT proceeds to join the facial nerve (FN).

    Taste sensation pathway from the anterior two-thirds of the tongue:
    - The taste sensation starts at the lingual nerve, a branch of the mandibular nerve (V3, which is the third branch of the trigeminal nerve).
    - The sensation is then carried by the CT to the facial nerve (FN).
    - From the FN, the signal goes to the geniculate ganglion (GG).
    - It then travels through the nervus intermedius to the nucleus solitarius, also known as the gustatory nucleus, in the brainstem.

14. **Where is the greater superficial petrosal nerve (GSPN), and what is its function?**
    - It is in the temporal bone, and the GSPN is relevant in mastoidectomy for its role in tear secretion. Surgeons must identify and preserve this nerve during surgery to prevent dry eye syndrome. It runs from the lacrimal gland to the geniculate ganglion, carrying parasympathetic secretomotor fibres.

    Greater superficial petrosal nerve (GSPN) pathway to the middle ear:
    - The GSPN enters the middle ear through the facial hiatus and connects with the facial nerve (FN) at the geniculate ganglion (GG).
    - Taste signals from the tonsillar fossa and palate are carried by the GSPN to the geniculate ganglion (GG).
    - From the GG, the signals travel through the nervus intermedius to the nucleus solitarius, also known as the gustatory nucleus, in the brainstem.

    Lacrimal gland innervation pathway:
    - The pathway begins at the superior salivatory nucleus, where signals travel through the nervus intermedius to reach the geniculate ganglion (GG).
    - From the GG, the greater superficial petrosal nerve (GSPN) passes through the facial hiatus, where it is joined by the deep petrosal nerve at the foramen lacerum. This junction provides sympathetic innervation.
    - The combined nerves form the vidian nerve, which travels through the vidian canal.
    - The vidian nerve then synapses in the sphenopalatine (pterygopalatine) ganglion.
    - From there, signals are conveyed via the superior maxillary nerve to the lacrimal gland, facilitating tear production.

15. **What is Jacobson's nerve, and what is its function?**

    Jacobson's nerve, or the tympanic branch of the glossopharyngeal nerve (CN IX), has a primary role in sensing changes in the middle ear's environment. It provides sensory innervation to the mucosa of the middle ear and mastoid air cells. Additionally, it contributes to the tympanic plexus, which plays a role in regulating blood flow within the middle ear. This function is crucial for maintaining the health and proper functioning of the middle ear structures. While not directly involved in hearing, Jacobson's nerve's integrity is essential for the overall health of the ear, as damage to it can lead to issues with pressure regulation and possibly ear infections.

16. **Are there any ways to avoid BIPP allergy?**

    In mastoidectomy, bismuth iodoform paraffin paste (BIPP) is used for packing. To avoid allergy, alternatives like antibiotic-impregnated gauze or synthetic packing materials can be used. Preoperative testing for BIPP sensitivity is recommended for at-risk patients to select the most appropriate packing material and prevent allergic reactions.

2.4 Stapedotomy

Indications for Surgery [4]

- Otosclerosis with conductive hearing loss >20 dB
- Stapes fixation due to other causes (e.g. congenital stapes fixation, tympanosclerosis)
- Failed previous stapes surgery

Specific Risks Involved with the Surgery [4]

- Bleeding
- Infection
- Hearing loss: dead ear (>1%)—sensorineural (1–5%) and conductive (5–15%)—or no significant improvement of hearing
- Tinnitus
- Vertigo or dizziness
- Perilymphatic fistula
- Facial nerve injury (rare)
- Taste disturbance (chorda tympani injury)
- Prosthesis malfunction: displacement, dislocation, protrusion, extrusion
- Reparative granuloma
- Late failure
- Need to abandon
- Tragal/endaural wound

Steps of the Surgery

1. Administration of local or general anaesthesia
2. Patient positioning: supine with the head turned to one side using head ring
3. Selection of the surgical approach (endaural or transcanal/permeatal)
4. Tympanomeatal flap elevation to expose the middle ear
5. Identification and preservation of the facial nerve, chorda tympani, and other critical structures
6. Removal of a small portion of the posterosuperior canal wall with a curette to fully expose stapes
7. Inspection and palpation of the ossicular chain, to confirm the diagnosis
8. Removal of the stapes superstructure and creation of a small hole in the footplate (stapedotomy) using a drill or laser. If too much force is applied or the hole is drilled too deeply, it can penetrate the vestibule, causing trauma to the cochlear structures and risking perilymphatic fluid leakage. This fluid imbalance in the inner ear can impair cochlear function and lead to sensorineural hearing loss.
9. Measurement and insertion of the stapes prosthesis and crimping to the incus as seen in Fig. 2.7
10. Graft placement (if necessary) to seal the oval window
11. Tympanomeatal flap repositioning and application of antibiotic ointment
12. Packing of the ear canal

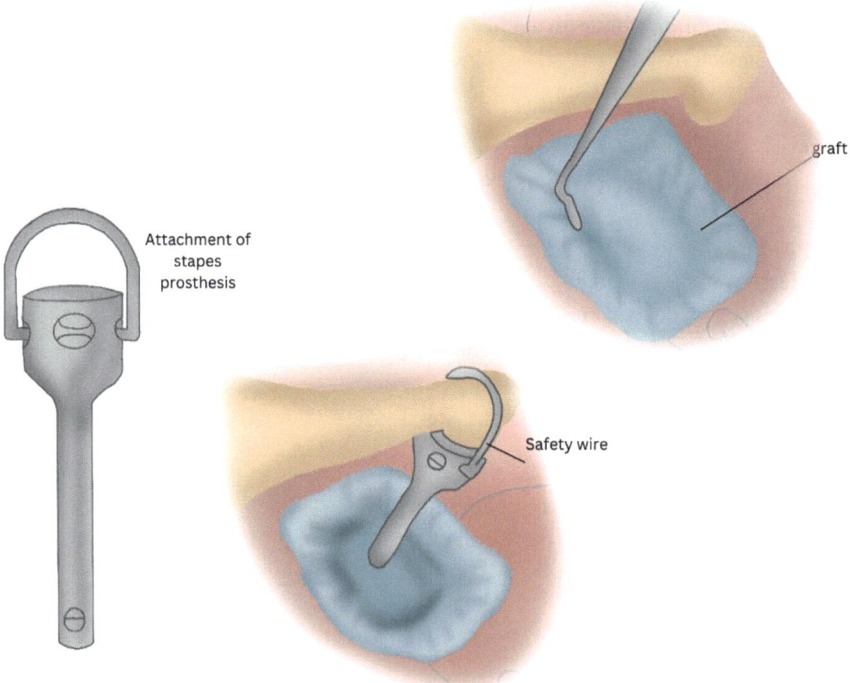

Fig. 2.7 Stapes prosthesis insertion with no stapes footplate. Illustrated by Vikum Liyanaarachchi

Important Points to Note During the Surgery

- Preserve the facial nerve, chorda tympani, and other critical structures.
- Avoid excessive manipulation of the ossicular chain and stapes footplate.
- Ensure proper sizing, positioning, and crimping of the stapes prosthesis.
- Prevent a perilymphatic fistula by sealing the oval window.

Questions a Consultant Might Ask a Trainee About the Operation

1. **What are the key differences between a stapedectomy and stapedotomy, and how do you decide which approach to use?**

   A stapedectomy involves the removal of the stapes footplate or part of it (as well as the superstructure), while a stapedotomy involves creating a small hole in the stapes footplate. Both are often followed by insertion of a piston prosthesis. Stapedotomy is generally preferred due to a lower risk of sensorineural hearing loss and better hearing outcomes [4]. However, the choice depends on the surgeon's experience and preference, as well as the specific patient anatomy and aetiology of stapes fixation. Stapedectomy is no longer performed, except in revision cases. Figure 2.8 shows a stapes footplate with stapedotomy—the piston will sit in this.

2. **What would you do if the footplate is fractured and there was leak of perilymph?**

   If steroid flood, proceed with piston insertion (some would advocate placing this on a vein graft), seal with fascia, then steroids, and antibiotics post-op.

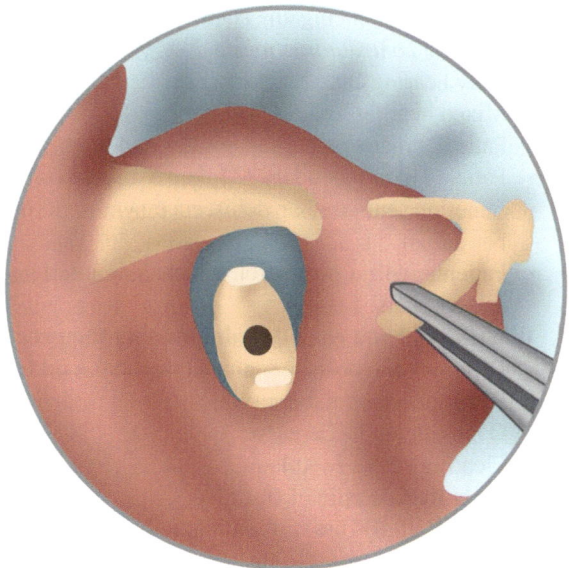

Fig. 2.8 Stapedotomy performed leaving the stapes footplate with a central hole for the piston to sit in. Illustrated by Vikum Liyanaarachchi

Inform the patient and follow up carefully with audiology. A perilymphatic leak can lead to a dead ear.

3. **What are the main goals of stapes surgery, and how do you determine if the surgery is successful?**

    The main goals of stapes surgery are to improve hearing by restoring ossicular chain mobility. The success of the surgery is determined by post-operative audiometric testing, which should demonstrate an improvement in conductive hearing loss and air-bone gap closure.

4. **What are some factors that may contribute to surgical failure or complications following stapes surgery?**

    Factors that may contribute to surgical failure or complications include improper sizing, positioning, or crimping of the stapes prosthesis; excessive manipulation of the ossicular chain; facial nerve or chorda tympani injury; perilymphatic fistula; and pre-existing sensorineural hearing loss.

5. **How do you manage a patient with persistent conductive hearing loss or sensorineural hearing loss after stapes surgery?**

    This implies that the stapes prosthesis is too short, or too long, respectively. For patients with persistent conductive hearing loss after stapes surgery, revision surgery may be considered to address issues with the stapes prosthesis. For patients with persistent or new-onset sensorineural hearing loss, options include hearing aids, cochlear implants (in cases of severe-to-profound sensorineural hearing loss), or bone conduction devices. The choice of management depends on the patient's preferences, the degree of hearing loss, and the cause of the hearing loss.

6. **What are the contraindications for stapedotomy surgery?**
    - *Absolute contraindication*:
    - Active infection in the middle or external ear which should be addressed first before commencing any stapes surgery [4]
    - *Relative contraindications*:
    - Only hearing ear.
    - Mixed hearing loss.
    - Patient's main concern is tinnitus and not hearing loss.
    - Patients with secondary Meniere's disease or with preoperative vertigo.
    - Superior semicircular dehiscence syndrome on CT (stapes surgery exacerbates this).
    - Patients with a profession which may interfere with the surgery, e.g. pilots and acrobats.

7. **When would you consider abandoning the procedure?**

    Different diagnosis, e.g. malleo-incudal joint fixation
    Persistent stapedial artery
    Overhanging facial nerve
    Floating stapes footplate

8. **What is Belfast rule of thumb?**

    Belfast 15/30 dB rule of thumb is to help identify which patients would benefit from reconstructive middle ear surgery. It states that a patient is likely to report a significant benefit if the post-operative hearing level can be improved to 30 dB or better and the interaural difference reduced to <15 dB.

2.5 Ossiculoplasty

Indications for Surgery [7]

- Conductive hearing loss resulting from ossicular chain discontinuity/loss/trauma

Specific Risks Involved with the Surgery [7]

- Bleeding
- Infection
- Hearing loss/failure: sensorineural (1–5%), conductive (5–15%)
- Tinnitus
- Vertigo or dizziness
- Facial nerve injury (rare)
- Taste disturbance (chorda tympani injury)
- Prosthesis malfunction: displacement, dislocation, protrusion, extrusion

Steps of the Surgery

1. Patient positioning: supine with the head turned to opposite side.
2. Administration of local or general anaesthesia.
3. Selection of the surgical approach (endaural, postauricular, or permeatal).
4. Tympanomeatal flap elevation to expose the tympanic membrane and middle ear.
5. Identification and preservation of the facial nerve, chorda tympani, and other critical structures.
6. Inspection of the ossicular chain to determine the site of disruption or dysfunction.
7. Removal of any diseased or eroded ossicles.
8. Reconstruction of the ossicular chain using autograft, allograft, or synthetic materials. Synthetic prostheses will need a disc of cartilage placed between the drum and the prosthesis to prevent extrusion through the drum. Alternatively, the malleus can be transposed posteriorly, and the prosthesis placed under this.
9. Assessment of ossicular chain mobility and function.
10. Tympanomeatal flap repositioning and application of antibiotic ointment.
11. Packing of the ear canal.

Important Points to Note During the Surgery

- Preserve the facial nerve, chorda tympani, and other critical structures.
- Minimize handling and manipulation of the middle ear structures to prevent scarring, adhesions, and post-operative complications.
- Choose the appropriate graft material and prosthesis type for the specific ossicular chain defect (e.g. partial ossicular replacement prosthesis [PORP] or total ossicular replacement prosthesis [TORP]).
- Ensure proper sizing, positioning, and stability of the prosthesis.
- Assess the mobility and function of the reconstructed ossicular chain to ensure optimal hearing outcomes.

Questions a Consultant Might Ask a Trainee About the Operation

1. **What are the different types of ossiculoplasty, and how do you decide which approach to use?**

    There are several types of ossiculoplasty, including type I (reconstruction of the incudostapedial joint, e.g. with bone cement), type II (incus interposition), type III (PORP), and type IV (TORP)—see Figs. 2.9 and 2.10. The choice of

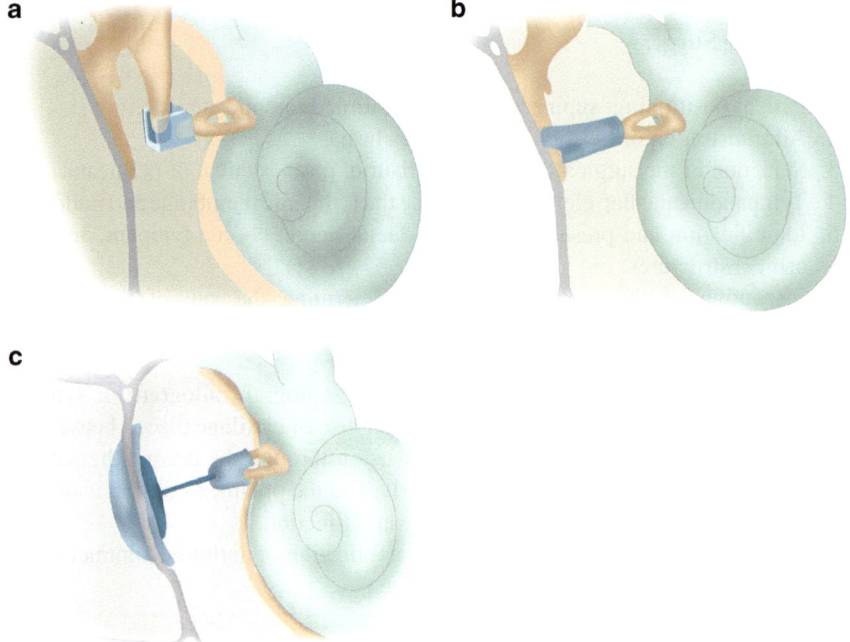

Fig. 2.9 Partial ossicular replacement prosthesis—three examples. (**a**) Applebaum prosthesis. (**b**) Crutch and cup prosthesis. (**c**) Classical PORP. Illustrated by Vikum Liyanaarachchi

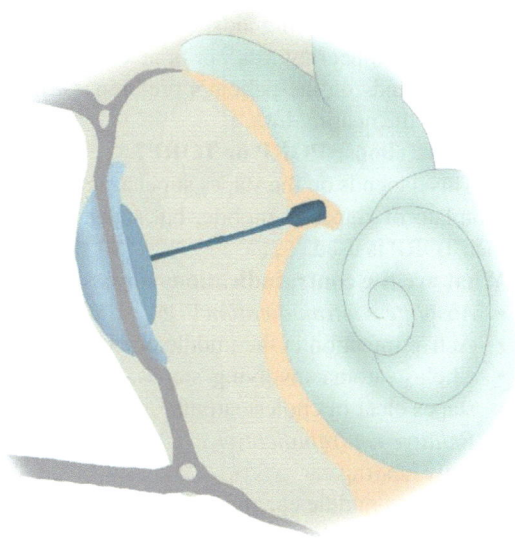

Fig. 2.10 Total ossicular replacement prosthesis (TORP). Illustrated by Vikum Liyanaarachchi

approach depends on the specific ossicular chain defect, the extent of the disease, and the surgeon's experience and preference [7].

2. **How do you minimize the risk of sensorineural hearing loss during ossiculoplasty?**

   To minimize the risk of sensorineural hearing loss, use gentle and controlled movements, avoid excessive force on the ossicular chain, and avoid excessive heat generation during drilling or use of a laser.

3. **What factors should be considered when selecting graft materials and prostheses for ossiculoplasty?**

   Factors to consider include biocompatibility, stability, risk of extrusion, potential for infection, availability, and cost. Autografts (e.g. cartilage, bone) have a lower risk of infection and extrusion compared to allografts and synthetic materials but may be limited in availability or size.

4. **What are some factors that may contribute to surgical failure or complications following ossiculoplasty?**

   Factors that may contribute to surgical failure or complications include improper sizing, positioning, or stability of the prosthesis; excessive manipulation of the ossicular chain; scarring or adhesions in the middle ear; Eustachian tube dysfunction; facial nerve or chorda tympani injury; and pre-existing sensorineural hearing loss.

5. **How do you manage a patient with persistent conductive hearing loss or sensorineural hearing loss after ossiculoplasty?**

   For patients with persistent conductive hearing loss after ossiculoplasty, revision surgery may be considered to address issues with the prosthesis, ossicular chain, or middle ear adhesions. Alternatively, a hearing aid should be consid-

ered. For patients with persistent or new-onset sensorineural hearing loss, options include hearing aids, cochlear implants (in cases of severe-to-profound sensorineural hearing loss), or bone conduction devices. The choice of management depends on the patient's preferences, the degree of hearing loss, and the cause of the hearing loss.
6. **When to choose PORP or TORP?**
   This depends on the stapes superstructure. If present, PORP could be used. If footplate of stapes is mobile, but superstructure is absent or partially eroded, then TORP is used.
7. **What are the contraindications for ossiculoplasty?**
   - *Absolute contraindication* [7]:
   - Active infection in the middle or external ear
   - Cholesteatoma involving stapes—staged reconstruction advised, i.e. when stapes clear of cholesteatoma
   - *Relative contraindications*:
   - Only hearing ear
   - Reduced middle ear space
   - Repeated surgical failures

2.6 Cochlear Implantation

Indications for Surgery [8]

- Severe-to-profound sensorineural hearing loss in one or both ears
- Limited benefit from hearing aids
- Congenital or acquired hearing loss that impacts speech perception and development

Specific Risks Involved with the Surgery [8]

- Bleeding
- Infection
- Facial nerve injury (rare)
- Meningitis (rare)
- Cerebrospinal fluid leakage (rare)
- Tinnitus
- Dizziness or vertigo
- Temporary altered taste (chorda tympani injury during posterior tympanotomy)
- Failure or malfunction of the implant
- Device migration or extrusion
- Loss of remaining hearing

2 Otology

Steps of the Surgery

1. Patient positioning: supine with the head turned to one side
2. Administration of general anaesthesia
3. Performed via a postauricular approach
4. Creation of a subperiosteal pocket or shallow cortical recess for the implant receiver/stimulator
5. Drilling of the mastoid cavity to include a posterior tympanotomy to expose the middle ear (mesotympanum)
6. Identification and preservation of the facial nerve, chorda tympani, and other critical structures
7. Cochleostomy: creation of a small opening in the cochlea or insertion through the round window (Fig. 2.11)
8. Insertion of the electrode array into the cochlea
9. Closure of the cochleostomy site with tissue or other materials to prevent cerebrospinal fluid leakage
10. Placement of the receiver/stimulator in the subperiosteal pocket/cortical recess and securing with sutures or bone anchors or bone wax

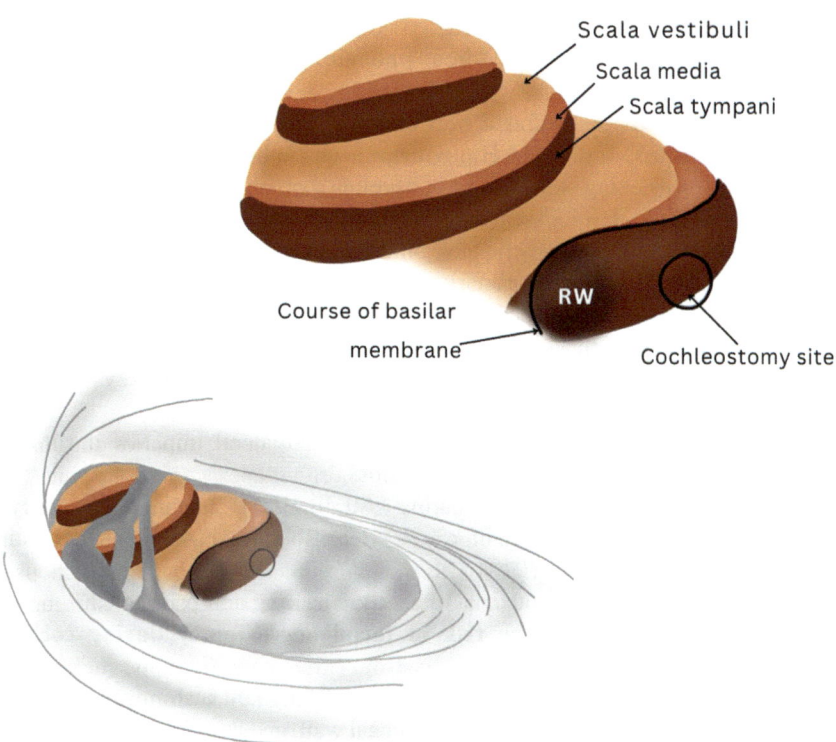

Fig. 2.11 Cochleostomy. Illustrated by Vikum Liyanaarachchi

11. Wound closure and application of a pressure dressing

Important Points to Note During the Surgery

- Preserve the facial nerve, chorda tympani, and other critical structures.
- Minimize drilling in the mastoid cavity to avoid damage to the inner ear structures and reduce the risk of complications.
- Perform atraumatic insertion of the electrode array into the cochlea to preserve residual hearing and minimize the risk of post-operative complications.
- Ensure proper positioning and stability of the implant components to prevent device migration or extrusion.
- Test the integrity and function of the implant intraoperatively to ensure optimal post-operative outcomes.

Questions a Consultant Might Ask a Trainee About the Operation

1. **What are the indications for cochlear implantation in the NHS as per the NICE guidelines (2019) [9]?.**
   Bilateral:
   - Pre-lingually deafened children who are offered simultaneous bilateral implants.
   - Bilateral severe-to-profound hearing loss (≥ 80 dB HL at two or more frequency at 0.5, 1, 2, 3, 4 kHz) without acoustic hearing whose speech, language, or listening skills have not developed or are not maintained at a level appropriate to developmental age and cognitive ability of the child.
   - Adults who are blind or who have other disabilities that increase their reliance on auditory stimuli as a primary sensory mechanism for spatial awareness.
   - Bilateral severe-to-profound hearing ≥ 80 dB HL (at 2 or more frequency at 0.5, 1, 2, 3, 4 kHz), a score of <50% Arthur Boothroyd (AB) sentence testing at a sound intensity of 70 dB SPL.

   Unilateral:
   - Post-lingually deafened adults are offered unilateral implants if suffering from further disability such as visual loss.
   - Bilateral severe-to-profound hearing ≥ 80 dB HL (at 2 or more frequency at 0.5, 1, 2, 3, 4 kHz), a score of <50% Arthur Boothroyd (AB) sentence testing at a sound intensity of 70 dB SPL.
   - Patients require a 3-month trial of acoustic hearing aids prior to CI.

2. **How do you minimize the risk of facial nerve injury during cochlear implantation?**
   To minimize the risk of injury, first identify the key anatomical landmarks, such as the sigmoid sinus, posterior ear canal wall, and lateral semicircular canal. Use a 4 mm diamond burr for drilling vertically (parallel to the underlying facial nerve) just behind the posterior canal wall, below the inferior edge of the lateral

SCC, and employ gentle and controlled movements. Constantly irrigate the area to reduce the risk of thermal injury. Watch for the nerve (light pink) or the tiny vessels that lie within its sheath. Monitoring the facial nerve function intraoperatively and using a facial nerve stimulator set to 0.5 mA can also be helpful.

3. **What are some factors that may affect the patient's post-operative performance with a cochlear implant?**

    Factors that may affect post-operative performance include the patient's age at implantation (pre- or post-lingually deaf), the duration of deafness, the aetiology of hearing loss, the degree of residual hearing, the choice of implant and electrode array, the quality of the surgical technique, and the patient's commitment to rehabilitation and follow-up care.

4. **What are some potential complications of cochlear implantation, and how can they be managed?**

    Potential complications include bleeding, infection, facial nerve injury, meningitis, cerebrospinal fluid leakage, tinnitus, dizziness or vertigo, failure or malfunction of the implant, and device migration or extrusion. Complications can be managed by using appropriate surgical techniques, intraoperative facial nerve monitoring, aseptic practices, post-operative care, and prompt intervention for any issues that arise.

5. **How do you manage a patient with a failed or malfunctioning cochlear implant?**

    If a cochlear implant fails or malfunctions, the first step is to perform a thorough diagnostic evaluation, including audiological testing, imaging, and device interrogation, to determine the cause of the problem. If the issue is related to the implant itself, revision surgery may be necessary to replace the malfunctioning component or the entire device. If the issue is related to programming or rehabilitation, adjustments can be made to the implant's settings or additional support can be provided to optimize the patient's outcomes.

6. **What are the components of the CI?**

    External Device:
    - Microphone (placed above ear)
    - Processor (placed behind the ear or worn)
    - Transmitter coil (directly overlies internal component via magnet)

    Implanted Device:
    - Receiver coil
    - Stimulator
    - Electrode array (placed in the **scala tympani** via a cochleostomy or the round window). Apical electrodes = low frequency. Basal electrodes = high frequency

    See Fig. 2.12.

7. **What are the different types of CI?**
    - Multichannel: Up to 22 electrode arrays.
    - Hybrid: Both electrical and acoustic mechanisms are used in patients with severe-to-profound high-frequency SNHL with relatively good low frequencies, so preserving apical cochlea function when inserting the electrode, and acoustic hearing aid can be used for the low frequencies. "Soft surgery" is

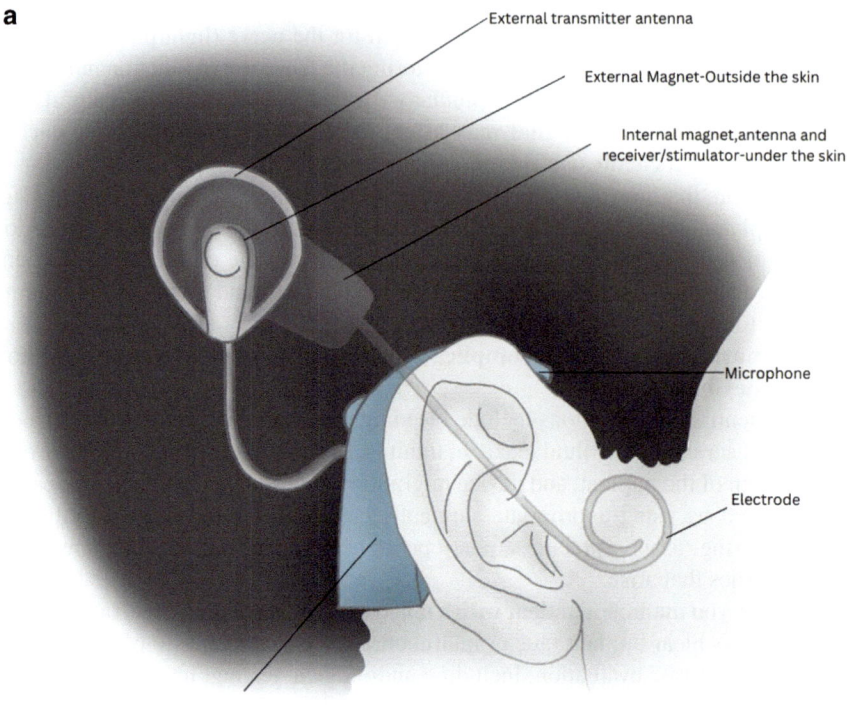
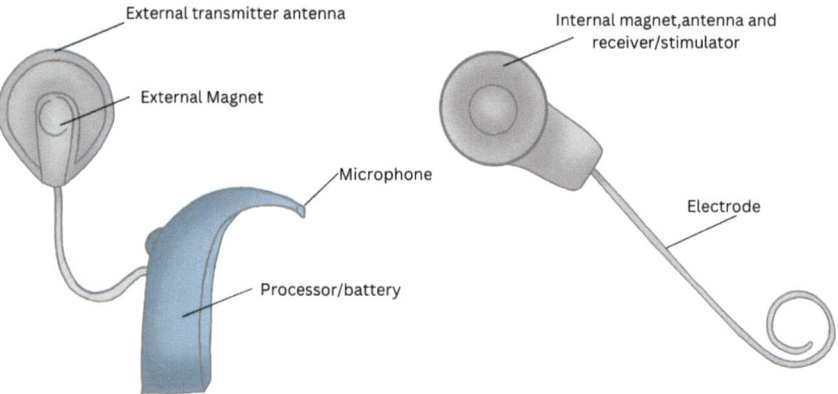

Fig. 2.12 Cochlear implant device. (**a**) shown in situ with sagittal view; (**b**) cochlear implant device shown and labelled. Illustrated by Vikum Liyanaarachchi

employed. This is the choice of a thinner, shorter electrode array that is modiolus hugging and inserted very slowly, following a steroid flood (dexamethasone solution to flood the middle and inner ear after the cochleostomy), with the intention of preserving any residual (low-frequency) hearing.
- Split (double) electrode: for cochlear anomalies such as labyrinthitis ossificans (e.g. following meningitis).

2.7 Labyrinthectomy

Indications for Surgery [10]

- Intractable Meniere's disease with severe vertigo attacks
- Other causes of incapacitating vertigo not responding to conservative management
- Patients with no useful hearing in the affected ear
- Access to the IAM

Specific Risks Involved with the Surgery [10]

- Bleeding
- Infection
- Hearing loss in the affected ear (complete)
- Dizziness or vertigo (temporary or persistent)
- Facial nerve injury (rare)
- Cerebrospinal fluid leakage (rare)

Steps of the Surgery

1. Patient positioning: supine with the head turned to one side
2. Administration of general anaesthesia
3. Drilling of the mastoid cavity to expose the labyrinth
4. Identification and preservation of the facial nerve, incus, and other critical structures
5. Removal of the semicircular canals while preserving the facial nerve
6. Packing of the labyrinthine cavity with bone pâté, fat, or other materials
7. Wound closure and application of a pressure dressing

Important Points to Note During the Surgery

- Preserve the facial nerve and other critical structures.
- Ensure complete removal of the labyrinthine structures to achieve optimal vertigo control.

- Prepare the patient for the possibility of post-operative imbalance, which may require vestibular rehabilitation, or preoperative transtympanic gentamicin injection, so the vertigo is not experienced at the same time as surgical recovery ("pre-hab").

Questions a Consultant Might Ask a Trainee About the Operation

1. **What is the main goal of labyrinthectomy, and how do you determine if the surgery is successful?**
    The main goal of labyrinthectomy is to control intractable vertigo by completely removing the labyrinthine structures. The success of the surgery is determined by the resolution of vertigo attacks and the patient's ability to regain balance through vestibular rehabilitation.
2. **How do you minimize the risk of facial nerve injury during labyrinthectomy?**
    To minimize the risk of facial nerve injury, identify key anatomical landmarks such as the facial nerve, incus, tegmen, and lateral semicircular canal. It may help to identify the horizontal/tympanic segment in the middle ear. When performing the labyrinthectomy, start drilling furthest away from the facial nerve, and slowly move anteriorly towards it. Use a facial nerve monitor intraoperatively to identify the facial nerve and avoid injury during drilling and labyrinth removal.
3. **What are some factors that may affect the patient's post-operative balance and recovery following labyrinthectomy?**
    Factors that may affect post-operative balance and recovery include the patient's age, general health, degree of preoperative vestibular dysfunction, quality of the surgical technique, and the patient's commitment to vestibular rehabilitation.
4. **What are some alternative surgical options for patients with intractable vertigo who are not candidates for labyrinthectomy?**
    Alternative surgical options for patients with intractable vertigo include endolymphatic sac decompression or shunt, vestibular nerve section, and chemical labyrinthectomy using intratympanic gentamicin injections. Triple-canal occlusion may also reduce the vertigo while preserving hearing.
5. **How do you manage a patient with persistent vertigo or imbalance following labyrinthectomy?**
    For patients with persistent vertigo or imbalance after labyrinthectomy, a thorough evaluation should be performed to rule out any underlying causes, such as incomplete labyrinth removal, complications, or central vestibular disorders. Vestibular rehabilitation therapy can be beneficial in helping patients regain balance and adapt to their new vestibular function. In some cases, additional surgical intervention may be necessary.
6. **What is Donaldson's line?**

Donaldson's line is an imaginary line drawn parallel to the horizontal/lateral semicircular canal that bisects the posterior semicircular canal. The endolymphatic sac will lie inferior to Donaldson's line.
7. **What is serviceable/non-serviceable hearing?**
    AAOHNS Criteria [11]:
    - **Serviceable Hearing:**
    (a) Class I: Speech discrimination score (SDS) 70–100% and PTA levels <30 dB
    (b) Class II: SDS 50–70% and PTA levels 30–50 dB
    - **Non-serviceable hearing:**
    (a) Class III: SDS 50–70% and PTA levels >50 dB
    (b) Class IV: SDS <50% any PTA

    A general rule of thumb is whether they can use a telephone on the affected side.

2.8   Vestibular Nerve Section

Indications for Surgery [12]

- **Vertigo control**: Aimed at patients suffering from severe, refractory vertigo due to Meniere's disease or other causes not amenable to conservative treatments.
- **Hearing consideration**: Ideally suited for individuals with serviceable hearing in the affected ear, where surgical intervention strives to maintain auditory function.
- **Vestibular schwannoma management**: Employed in the nuanced management of vestibular schwannomas, focusing on alleviating symptoms while aiming for tumour reduction or removal, mindful of preserving neural functionality.

Specific Risks Involved with the Surgery [12]

- Bleeding
- Infection
- Hearing loss in the affected ear (possible)
- Dizziness or vertigo (temporary or persistent)
- Facial nerve injury (rare)
- Cerebrospinal fluid leakage (rare)
- Meningitis (rare)
- Failure/non-resolution of symptoms

Steps of the Surgery

1. **Patient set-up**: Place the patient in a supine position, adjusting the head to be slightly elevated and rotated away from the side of surgery.

2. **Anaesthesia and safety measures**: Begin with the administration of general anaesthesia, complemented by the prophylactic use of antibiotics to ward off post-operative infections. The use of facial nerve monitoring is essential. Perioperative mannitol to reduce CSF pressure:
    - Additionally, deploying electrocochleography (ECoG) or brainstem auditory evoked responses (BAERs) can be invaluable for monitoring cochlear nerve function, providing a comprehensive safety net for critical neural structures.
3. **Surgical approach selection:**
    - **Middle fossa approach**: Best suited for patients with small tumours confined to the internal auditory canal and those with preserved hearing. This approach allows direct access to the canal without necessitating significant manipulation of the cerebellum or brainstem.
    - **Retrosigmoid approach:** Ideal for larger tumours that extend into the cerebellopontine angle. It offers a balance between good tumour visibility and hearing preservation, making it a versatile choice for a broad range of tumour sizes (Fig. 2.13).
    - **Translabyrinthine approach:** Preferred for patients with non-serviceable hearing or large tumours where hearing preservation is not a concern. This approach provides the most direct access to the tumour and the facial nerve, facilitating easier tumour removal but at the expense of hearing. Complete skeletonization of the middle fossa dura and sigmoid is required to optimize access.

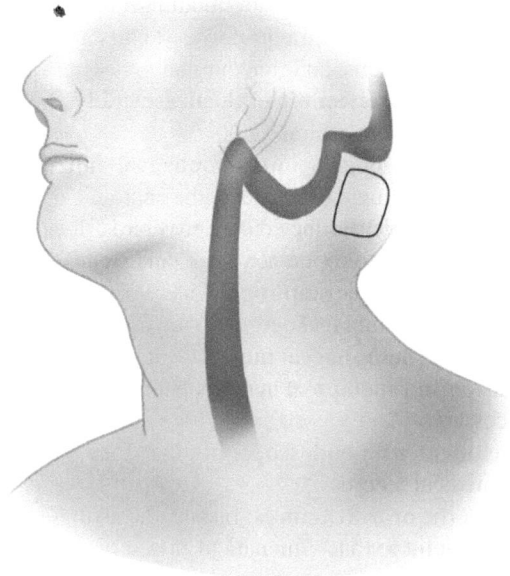

Fig. 2.13 Example of retrosigmoid approach. Illustrated by Vikum Liyanaarachchi

Decision-making factors include the tumour's size and extension, the patient's hearing status, and anatomical variations. Consideration of the patient's overall health, previous treatments, and specific goals for surgery (e.g. hearing preservation vs. complete tumour removal) also guide approach selection.

4. **Vestibular nerve isolation and sectioning:**
   - Microsurgical techniques are employed to carefully isolate the vestibular nerve. Intraoperative nerve stimulation confirms its identity, ensuring that the cochlear and facial nerves are preserved. This step is critical for maintaining hearing and facial muscle function.
   - The vestibular nerve is then sectioned with precision, using either microscissors or a laser, under high magnification to ensure a clean cut and to minimize the risk of damaging adjacent structures.

5. **Surgical Closure and Recovery:**

   Before closure, meticulous inspection for bleeding is performed, using bipolar cautery or applying haemostatic agents to ensure complete haemostasis. This step is vital to prevent post-operative haematoma formation.

   The operative site is closed in layers, using absorbable sutures for the deeper layers and skin adhesive or sutures for the skin layer. Abdominal fat is used to pack the mastoid cavity. A sterile, pressure dressing is applied to support healing and minimize swelling.

   Post-operative care includes close monitoring for signs of facial nerve dysfunction and infection, along with a regimen for pain management and antibiotic continuation. The patient is scheduled for follow-up visits for wound inspection, hearing tests, and facial nerve function assessment, ensuring a comprehensive recovery plan.

   Important points to note during the surgery:
   - Preserve the facial nerve, cochlear nerve, and other critical structures.
   - Minimize damage to surrounding structures during drilling and dissection.
   - Ensure complete sectioning of the vestibular nerve to achieve optimal vertigo control.
   - Prepare the patient for the possibility of post-operative imbalance, which may require vestibular rehabilitation (or pre-habilitation, as above).

Questions a Consultant Might Ask a Trainee About the Operation

1. **What is the main goal of vestibular nerve section, and how do you determine if the surgery is successful?**

   The main goal of vestibular nerve section is to control intractable vertigo by selectively cutting the vestibular nerve while preserving hearing. The success of the surgery is determined by the resolution of vertigo attacks and the patient's ability to regain balance through vestibular rehabilitation.

2. **How do you minimize the risk of facial nerve injury during vestibular nerve section?**

To minimize the risk of facial nerve injury, identify key anatomical landmarks such as the facial nerve, cochlear nerve, and internal auditory canal. Use a facial nerve monitor intraoperatively to identify the facial nerve and avoid injury during drilling and nerve sectioning.

3. **What are the differences between the middle fossa, retrosigmoid, and translabyrinthine approaches to vestibular nerve section, and how do you choose the most appropriate approach?**

   The middle fossa approach provides a direct view of the IAC and is better suited for patients with good hearing.

   The retrosigmoid approach is a more posterior approach to the IAC, which is preferred in patients with small or absent mastoid air cells.

   The translabyrinthine approach involves the removal of the labyrinth and is best for patients with no useful hearing in the affected ear. The choice of approach depends on the patient's hearing status, the surgeon's experience, and the specific anatomy of the patient.

4. **What are some alternative surgical options for patients with intractable vertigo who are not candidates for vestibular nerve section?**

   Alternative surgical options for patients with intractable vertigo include endolymphatic sac decompression or shunt, labyrinthectomy (for patients with no useful hearing), and chemical labyrinthectomy using intratympanic gentamicin injections. Triple-canal occlusion may also reduce the vertigo while preserving hearing.

5. **How do you manage a patient with persistent vertigo or imbalance following vestibular nerve section?**

   For patients with persistent vertigo or imbalance after vestibular nerve section, a thorough evaluation should be performed to rule out any underlying causes, such as incomplete nerve section, complications, or central vestibular disorders.

6. **What is Trautman's triangle?**

   Recognizing Trautman's triangle is pivotal for navigating the retrosigmoid approach, offering a landmark that helps safely guide the surgeon towards the posterior fossa. It is clear demarcation to assist in avoiding vital structures such as the sigmoid sinus and the labyrinth, crucial for minimizing risk and enhancing surgical safety. It is bounded superiorly by the superior petrosal sinus, inferiorly by the sigmoid sinus, and anteriorly by the bony labyrinth [11].

7. **How are the nerves at the internal auditory canal (IAC) arranged?**

   The nerves are divided by Bill's bar (vertical crest) and falciform crest (horizontal crest) into three sections: facial nerve and nervus intermedius are anterosuperior, and superior vestibular nerve posterosuperior. Cochlear nerve is anteroinferior, and inferior vestibular nerve posteroinferior. The acronym to help remember this is 7-up and Coke-down—referring to the seventh cranial nerve being anterosuperior and cochlear nerve anteroinferior.

8. **What is singular nerve neurectomy?**

   It is the division of singular nerve (posterior ampullary nerve) which is a branch of inferior vestibular nerve and supplies posterior semicircular canal.

This targeted procedure, reserved for intractable BPPV affecting the posterior semicircular canal, demonstrates the surgical precision required for vestibular nerve section.

2.9 Bone-Anchored Hearing Aids (BAHAs)

Indications for Surgery [13]

- Conductive hearing loss:
  - Middle ear conditions where conventional hearing aids are ineffective, such as chronic ear infections or anatomical abnormalities
  - Patients with skin issues or allergies that prevent the use of traditional hearing aids
- Sensorineural hearing loss:
  - Single-sided deafness (SSD) where one ear has profound hearing loss while the other has normal hearing

Specific Risks Involved with the Surgery [13]

- Infection at the surgery site
- Skin irritation or wound healing problems around the abutment + skin overgrowth
- Failure of the osseointegration process (where the bone does not bond to the implant properly)
- Possibility of numbness around the implant area
- Chronic pain
- Damage to dura
- Bleeding (sigmoid sinus)

Steps of the Surgery

1. Assessment and planning: Detailed audiological evaluation and physical examination to assess suitability for BAHA.
2. Anaesthesia administration: Procedure performed under general anaesthesia but can also be performed under local anaesthetic.
3. Shave patients' hair as required.
4. Mark the initial location—classically 50–55 mm posterior to external auditory canal and 10–15 mm superior to the superior attachment of the pinna (superior to linea temporalis).
5. Skin thickness is measured where the implant is placed. You may use a blue needle (dipped in methyl blue) to gage the depth (typically 3–4 mm) and also to mark the position for the drill.

6. A small incision made behind the ear over the region down to bone. Soft tissue is raised off the skull surface.
7. A countersink hole is drilled into the skull using a guide. The hole is then checked for complications such as bleeding or CSF leak. Then using a low-speed drill, a titanium implant is inserted.
8. Osseointegration period: A healing period of several weeks to months is allowed for the bone to bond with the implant.
9. Attachment of the abutment: Once osseointegration is confirmed, the abutment is attached to the implant.
10. Fitting of the sound processor: The external component is attached to the abutment; adjustments and programming are done for optimal hearing. See Fig. 2.14 to view in situ.

Important Points to Note During the Surgery

- Careful handling of the soft tissue to reduce the risk of infection and promote better healing
- Precise positioning of the implant to ensure the best possible sound transmission
- Monitoring for any signs of adverse reactions or complications during the osseointegration period

Questions a Consultant Might Ask a Trainee About the Operation

1. **What advantages does a BAHA offer over traditional hearing aids?**

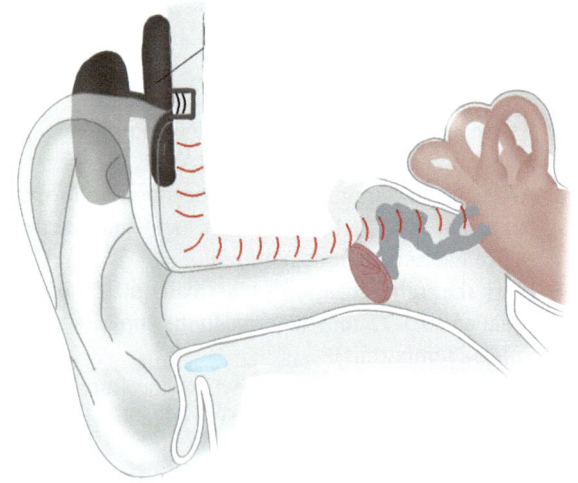

Fig. 2.14 Bone-anchored hearing aid in situ. Illustrated by Vikum Liyanaarachchi

BAHAs bypass problems in the outer or middle ear by directly stimulating the cochlea, offering clearer sound quality. They are particularly beneficial for patients who cannot wear traditional hearing aids due to otorrhoea, recurrent infections, skin allergies, or anatomical issues.

2. **How long does the osseointegration process take?**

    The osseointegration process typically takes several weeks to a few months, depending on factors like the patient's age and bone quality [13].

3. **Can BAHAs be used in children?**

    A3: Yes, BAHAs are an effective option for children with congenital ear defects or chronic ear infections who are unsuitable for conventional hearing aids.

4. **Is the BAHA surgery reversible?**

    If necessary, the implant can be removed. The bone at the implant site usually heals and fills in post-removal.

5. **How does a patient care for their BAHA post-surgery?**

    Care involves regular cleaning of the abutment site, monitoring for signs of infection or irritation, and routine visits to the audiologist for check-ups and adjustments.

6. **What exactly is osseointegration in the context of BAHA surgery?**

    Osseointegration refers to the process where the titanium implant bonds with the bone in the skull. This biological integration is crucial for the stability of the BAHA, as it provides a firm foundation for the sound processor. The titanium implants are usually coated with hydroxyapatite at manufacture to encourage osseointegration.

7. **What are the components that make up a BAHA system?**

    A BAHA system comprises three main parts: the titanium implant that is inserted into the skull bone, the abutment that connects the implant to the external component, and the sound processor, which is the external device capturing and processing sound. The processor transmits sound vibrations through the abutment to the implant, which then directs them to the cochlea via bone conduction.

8. **How can you classify bone conduction hearing aids?**

    Direct drive (less skin and soft tissue attenuation and less physical sensation of the device):
    - Percutaneous, e.g. Ponto and BAHA
    - Active transcutaneous implanted transducer: e.g. Bonebridge™

    Skin drive:
    - Conventional (on eyeglasses or softband)
    - Passive transcutaneous implanted magnet, e.g. Sophono™ and BAHA Attract™

    In the mouth:
    - SoundBite

9. **What are the audiological criteria for BAHA?**

    Birmingham criteria:

- **PTA**: Average bone conduction thresholds (0.5–4 kHz) <45 dB HL (ear level) and <55 dB HL (for body worn) in the better hearing ear. However, newer BAHA units can be used even with a 65 dB SNHL (BAHA 5 superpower sound processor).
- Speech discrimination score >60%.

  Reasonable expectations and social support must be considered when choosing candidates for BAHA.

10. **What are the contraindications for BAHA?**
    - Audiological: PTA **BC thresholds** (0.5–3.0 kHz) worse than 55 dB HL, SD <65%—however, with newer models/sound processors, this can change [13].
    - Age <4 years (thin bone).
    - Skin disease: eczema, psoriasis.
    - Bone diseases: Paget's disease or osteogenesis imperfecta.
    - Poor compliance or social support.
11. **What is the alterative to BAHA in patients with single-sided SNHL?**

    CROS: Contralateral routing of signal aid, cochlear implant (if funded)
12. **What classification is there for post-operative BAHA skin complications?**

    Holger classification:
    - Grade 0: no skin reaction
    - Grade I: redness with slight swellings
    - Grade II: redness with moderate swelling
    - Grade III: redness with moderate swelling and granulation tissues
    - Grade IV: profound infection

    Grades I and II: local wound care +/− topical antibiotics and using of the healing cap

    Grade III: + removal of granulation tissues

    Grade IV: + removal of the device

References

1. Lous J, Burton MJ, Felding J, Ovesen T, Rovers M, Williamson I. Grommets (ventilation tubes) for hearing loss associated with otitis media with effusion in children. Cochrane Database Syst Rev. 2005;(1):CD001801.
2. National Institute for Health and Care Excellence (NICE). Otitis media with effusion in under 12s. NICE guideline [NG233]. 2023 Aug 30. Available from: https://www.nice.org.uk/guidance/ng233
3. Rosenfeld RM, Schwartz SR, Pynnonen MA, et al. Clinical practice guideline: tympanostomy tubes in children. Otolaryngol Head Neck Surg. 2013;149(1_suppl):S1–S35.
4. Fisch U, May JS, Linder T. Tympanoplasty, mastoidectomy, and stapes surgery. 2nd ed. New York: Thieme; 2008.
5. Ryu NG, Kim J. How to avoid facial nerve injury in mastoidectomy? J Audiol Otol. 2016;20(2):68.
6. Tan HE, Santa Maria PL, Eikelboom RH, Anandacoomaraswamy KS, Atlas MD. Type I tympanoplasty meta-analysis: a single variable analysis. Otol Neurotol. 2016;37(7):838–46.
7. Javia LR, Ruckenstein MJ. Ossiculoplasty. Otolaryngol Clin N Am. 2006;39(6):1177–89.

8. Deep NL, Dowling EM, Jethanamest D, Carlson ML. Cochlear implantation: an overview. J Neurol Surg B Skull Base. 2019;80(02):169–77.
9. National Institute for Health and Care Excellence (NICE). Cochlear implants for children and adults with severe to profound deafness. NICE technology appraisal guidance [TA566]. 2019 Jan 4. Available from: https://www.nice.org.uk/guidance/ta566
10. Sykopetrites V, Giannuzzi AL, Lauda L, Di Rubbo V, Bassi M, Sanna M. Surgical labyrinthectomy and cochlear implantation in Meniere's disease. Otol Neurotol. 2020;41(6):775–81.
11. American Academy of Otolaryngology-Head and Neck Surgery Foundation. Clinical practice guideline: sudden hearing loss (update). Otolaryngol Head Neck Surg. 2019;161(1_suppl):S1–S45. https://doi.org/10.1177/0194599819859885.
12. Silverstein H, Jackson LE. Vestibular nerve section. Otolaryngol Clin N Am. 2002;35(3):655–73.
13. Cass SP, Mudd PA. Bone-anchored hearing devices: indications, outcomes, and the linear surgical technique. Oper Tech Otolaryngol Head Neck Surg. 2010;21(3):197–206.

Rhinology

Carl van Wyk, Zohaib Siddiqui, Basim Wahba, and Keli Dusu

3.1 Functional Endoscopic Sinus Surgery (FESS)

Indications for surgery [1]:

- Chronic rhinosinusitis refractory to medical treatment
- Recurrent acute rhinosinusitis
- Sinusitis with complications such as orbital or intracranial extension
- Nasal polyps causing obstruction or recurrent infections
- Mucocele or pyocele of the paranasal sinuses
- Cerebrospinal fluid leaks or encephaloceles related to the paranasal sinuses
- Sinus and nasal tumours or masses
- Fungal sinusitis
- Endoscopic management of epistaxis
- Endoscopic dacrocystorhinostomy (DCR) as part of the management of epiphora
- Extended endoscopic approaches to the orbit, anterior skull base, or pituitary

Specific risks involved with the surgery [1]:

- Bleeding.
- Infection.
- Scarring or adhesions in the nasal cavity.

C. van Wyk (✉) · K. Dusu
Frimley Park Hospital, Camberley, UK
e-mail: frederik.vanwyk@nhs.net

Z. Siddiqui
Medway NHS Foundation Trust, Gillingham, Kent, UK

B. Wahba
Queen Victoria Hospital, East Grinstead, UK

© The Author(s), under exclusive license to Springer Nature Switzerland AG 2024
Z. Siddiqui et al. (eds.), *Essentials of ENT Surgical Procedures*,
https://doi.org/10.1007/978-3-031-71394-1_3

- Epiphora.
- Olfactory disturbance or loss.
- Injury to the orbit (common) may lead to surgical emphysema on blowing the nose (usually self-limiting).
- Injury to the orbital muscles may lead to diplopia.
- Injury to the eye (rare) may lead to vision loss/complete loss of sight (1:1000 cases).
- Injury to the skull base with cerebrospinal fluid leakage (1:1000 cases).
- Meningitis.
- Intracranial complications.

Prior to operating:

Review the computed tomography (CT) scans preoperatively to assess the sinus anatomy, paying particular attention to the osteomeatal complex and the frontal recess.

The **CLOSED** formula helps in identifying critical areas such as:

1. **C**ribriform plate height
2. **L**amina papyracea integrity
3. **O**ptic nerve, **O**rbit, and **O**nodi cells,
4. **S**phenoid sinus
5. Anterior **E**thmoidal artery and ethmoidal roof
6. CT **D**ental assessment

Steps of the surgery:

1. General anaesthesia is used. Total intravenous anaesthesia (TIVA) is preferred for reducing intraoperative/post-operative bleeding. Prepare the nasal cavity with topical decongestants to reduce mucosal bleeding.
2. Place the patient in a supine position with the head elevated (reverse Trendelenburg) at a 30° angle to reduce venous pressure and bleeding. Ensure that the face is fully visible to the surgeon for orientation and access. Eyelids can be taped shut on their lateral aspect as long as the eyes can be easily opened during surgery if needed.
3. Apply topical decongestants/vasoconstrictors to reduce mucosal swelling. This aids in better visualization and reduces the risk of mucosal damage during instrumentation, i.e. Moffett's solution (cocaine, adrenaline, 2 mL 1% bicarbonate, and sodium chloride). Modified Moffett's solution is often used in practice (100 mg cocaine hydrochloride, 1 mg of adrenaline in 10 mL of saline).
4. Drape the patient appropriately while keeping the eyes exposed for continuous monitoring. Avoid covering the mouth with drapes that would conceal bleeding from the mouth during surgery. The nostrils should be accessible for endoscopic entry and manipulation.
5. The patient should be positioned supine on the operating table with their head elevated at about 15°–30°. This head-up position helps reduce venous pressure

and minimize bleeding. The patient's head should be stabilized with a headrest, and the surgeon should ensure proper alignment to provide optimal access to the nasal structures.
6. Introduce a 0° or 30° endoscope gently into the nasal cavity. Survey the internal nasal anatomy, identifying key landmarks such as the inferior turbinate, middle turbinate, and septum. A 3-pass technique can be used; a 3-pass technique is where the endoscope is advanced along the nasal floor, along the middle meatus, between the inferior turbinate and middle turbinate, and superiorly, along superior turbinate/skull base (medial to the middle turbinate, but higher up, anatomy permitting).
7. Medialize the middle turbinate, taking care to preserve it if removal is not required.
8. **Uncinectomy**: Carefully perform an uncinectomy to access the maxillary ostium. This step requires precise dissection to avoid orbital damage while following the attachment superiorly, which will be a guide to the frontal recess. This can be performed in many ways, for example, using a curved instrument to fracture the uncinate and then remove it using a sharp or grasping instrument.
9. **Maxillary antrostomy**: Enlarge the natural maxillary ostium to improve sinus ventilation and drainage. Ensure the preservation of the mucociliary function by minimizing mucosal trauma. This can be performed with different instruments including a backbiter, a straight-through biter, a down biter, and debrider. Note that the debrider should not be used in the maxillary sinus area without first confirming that the maxillary sinus has been entered. This is due to the risk of entering the orbit in cases of maxillary hypoplasia such as silent sinus syndrome.
10. **Anterior ethmoidectomy**: Identify and start with the bulla ethmoidalis, "uncapping the egg", starting medially/inferiorly. Dissect the anterior ethmoid air cells with care to avoid the orbit laterally and the skull base superiorly. This can be performed with a microdebrider or an antrum curette. Identification of the anterior ethmoid artery is crucial to prevent severe bleeding (identification on the pre-op CT scan and maintaining surgical situational awareness will limit the risk of damage to the anterior ethmoidal artery).
11. **Posterior ethmoidectomy**: Identify the basal lamella of the middle turbinate. Proceed through the lamella lower (inferior) than the roof of the maxillary sinus. Dissect the posterior ethmoid air cells, maintaining spatial orientation to prevent injury, being conscious of the optic nerve being lateral and skull base superiorly. (Stay safe by identification of the skull base, be aware of sphenoethmoidal cells, and make sure that the lamina is intact on the preoperative CT scan of the sinuses.)
12. **Sphenoidotomy**: Perform a sphenoidotomy, if indicated, considering the sphenoid sinus's proximity to vital structures such as the internal carotid arteries and optic nerves. If possible, identify the sphenoid ostium. The safest point of entry will be medial and about 1 cm up from the posterior choana.
13. **Frontal sinusotomy**: If required, create a pathway to the frontal sinuses, which can be challenging due to their variable anatomy. The upper attachment of the

uncinate will help guide to the frontal recess. Techniques such as the use of balloon sinuplasty or the Draf procedures may be employed depending on the extent of disease and anatomy.
14. **Polyp removal and other interventions**: Address polyps or other pathological tissues encountered during the surgery, using microdebrider or other instruments as necessary for precise removal.
15. **Haemostasis and closure**: Achieve haemostasis to prevent post-operative bleeding. Adrenaline-soaked patties are useful during the operation to cause vasoconstriction and reduce bleeding. Packing may be placed, if necessary, although many surgeons now opt for absorbable materials or no packing at all to enhance patient comfort post-operatively.

Important points to note during the surgery:

- Identify key anatomical landmarks such as the middle turbinate, uncinate process attachment, ethmoid bulla, and face of sphenoid (consistent landmarks in sinus surgery are uncinate process, face of bulla, basal lamella, and face of sphenoid). See Fig. 3.1 for coronal view.

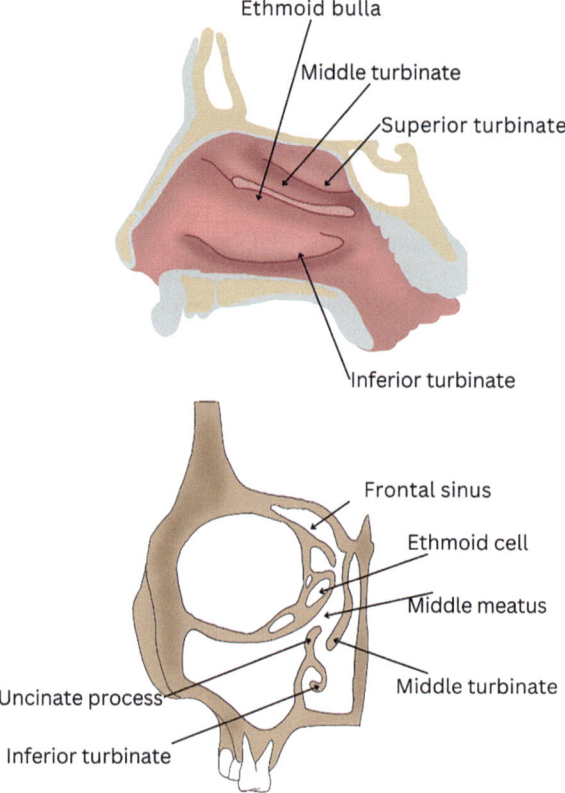

Fig. 3.1 Coronal view of sinus anatomy. (Illustrated by Vikum Liyanaarachchi)

- Use atraumatic techniques (such as through-cut instruments, debrider) to avoid injury to the mucosa and underlying structures.
- When operating near the orbits (lamina, ethmoidectomy), remember to check the eyes externally and ballot the eye to assess its location endoscopically to avoid injury.
- Achieve adequate exposure and access to the paranasal sinuses to facilitate complete treatment of the underlying pathology by good vasoconstriction.
- Monitor for complications such as orbital injury, skull base injury, or excessive bleeding. Always maintain situational awareness/spatial orientation.
- Carefully evaluate the preoperative CT scan, considering the CLOSED formula (Cribriform plate, Lamina papyracea, Orbit, Sphenoid sinus, Ethmoid roof, Dental roots) and Keros classification (for olfactory fossa depth) to assess the risk of complications and guide surgical planning.
- A septoplasty may be performed for access to the sinuses.

Questions a consultant might ask a trainee about the operation:

1. **What are the key anatomical landmarks to identify during FESS?**
   Key anatomical landmarks include the middle turbinate, uncinate process, ethmoid bulla, basal lamella, maxillary sinus, face of the sphenoid, and frontal recess [1].
2. **How do you minimize the risk of orbital injury during FESS?**
   To minimize the risk of orbital injury, the surgeon needs to have a sound understanding of the anatomy, study the CT scan for anatomical variations and defects of the lamina, and maintain situational awareness. The use of good vasoconstriction, atraumatic technique, and regular ballot of the eye will aid this. The orbit is at risk of injury when performing an uncinectomy, middle meatal antrostomy, and anterior and posterior ethmoidectomy.
3. **How do you manage a cerebrospinal fluid leak during FESS?**
   In the case of an intraoperative cerebrospinal fluid (CSF) leak, identify the site of the leak and repair it using a multi-layer closure technique, which may include the use of autologous (e.g. a fat plug, fascia lata) or synthetic materials, tissue glue, or a pedicled mucosal flap. Post-operatively, the patient should be monitored closely for signs of meningitis or recurrent CSF leakage.
4. **What is the importance of the CLOSED formula and Keros classification in preoperative CT scan evaluation for FESS, and how do they impact surgical planning?**
   The CLOSED formula (Cribriform plate, Lamina papyracea, Orbit, Sphenoid sinus, Ethmoid roof, Dental roots) and Keros classification (for olfactory fossa depth) are helpful for assessing the patient's unique anatomical variations, which can impact the risk of complications and the surgical approach. By identifying these variations, surgeons can plan the procedure more safely and be prepared to address any potential difficulties, reducing the risk of complications and improving surgical outcomes (insert drawing with Keros depths shown here or lower down).

5. **What is the importance of identifying anterior ethmoidal artery on the CT?**

    It is important to look for "Kennedy's nipple" sign if present, which shows the emergence of the anterior ethmoidal artery from the orbit running in a mesentery (not bone) free from the skull base. In these cases, there is a higher risk of injury of the artery leading to significant bleeding and a risk of bleeding into the orbit if the damaged vessel retracts into the orbit.

6. **What is the Keros classification?**

    The Keros classification is a method of classifying the depth of the olfactory fossa based on the height of the lateral lamella of the cribriform plate [1]. The Keros classification is used to evaluate the depth of the olfactory fossa and is important in surgical procedures as this will help guide you in FESS to avoid injury to the cribriform plate (base of skull).

    Type 1 olfactory fossa 1–3 mm deep
    Type 2 olfactory fossa 4–7 mm deep
    Type 3 olfactory fossa 8–16 mm
    Type 4 olfactory fossa with asymmetric skull base

7. **How can you differentiate between a sphenoethmoidal (Onodi) cell and the sphenoid sinus?**
    - Location: A sphenoethmoidal cell is an ethmoidal air cell extending superolateral to the sphenoid sinus, located above the sphenoid and in continuity with the posterior ethmoidal cells. The sphenoid sinus is below the sphenoethmoidal cell.
    - Identification on CT: Use coronal views to locate an air cell above the sphenoid. Confirm with axial and sagittal planes. Sphenoethmoidal cells are typically found above the roof of the maxillary sinus, while the sphenoid sinus is below.
    - Distance from nasal sill: The distance between the nasal sill and the sphenoid sinus is about 7 cm.
    - Optic canal bulge: In about 50% of cases, a sphenoethmoidal cell may show an optic canal bulge.
    - Natural ostium identification: Instead of following the posterior ethmoids to the sphenoid, identify the natural ostium to the sphenoid sinus through the intranasal approach (medial to the middle turbinate, 1 cm up from the posterior choana).

8. **What are the different types of superior attachment of the uncinate process?**
    - Type 1: insertion into the lamina papyracea (LP) (commonest, about 50%).
    - Type 2: insertion into an agger nasi cell.
    - Type 3: insertion into the lamina papyracea and junction of the middle turbinate with the cribriform plate.
    - Type 4: insertion into the junction of the middle turbinate with the cribriform plate.
    - Type 5: insertion into the ethmoid skull base.
    - Type 6: insertion into the middle turbinate.
    - Types of frontal sinus outflow due to varied superior uncinate attachment:

Table 3.1 Different types of frontal sinus surgery/Draf procedures

Draf I	Draf IIA	Draf IIB	Draf III (modified Lothrop)
The frontal recess and frontal infundibulum are cleared by removing the superior portion of the uncinate process, anterior ethmoid cells and cells within the frontal recess (agger nasi is preserved)	All cells within the frontal recess lateral to the middle turbinate attachment are opened in addition to the structures cleared in a Draf I procedure to directly open in the internal frontal sinus ostium	Extension of the Draf 2A procedure to include the entire ipsilateral floor of the frontal sinus including removing the middle turbinate attachment to the frontal sinus floor and extending the dissection medially to the nasal septum and intersinus septum (medial limit of dissection)	Creates a single common drainage pathway for the bilateral frontal sinuses. The structures cleared by bilateral Draf IIB are joined by removing the intersinus septum and superior nasal septum

See Fig. 3.2 for visualization of Draf procedures

- To lamina papyracea: results in a recessus terminalis. Frontal sinus outflow is into the middle meatus.
- To skull base: frontal sinus outflow is into the ethmoid infundibulum.
- To middle turbinate: frontal sinus outflow is into the ethmoid infundibulum.

9. **How do you prepare Moffett's solution?**

    To prepare Moffett's solution, mix 1 mL of adrenaline (1:1000), add 1–2 mL of cocaine (10%), and 2 mL of sodium bicarbonate (8.4%). Dilute the mixture in 5 mL of 0.9% NaCl saline, resulting in a total volume of 10 mL.

10. **What is image guidance/surgical navigation?**

    Image guidance, or surgical navigation, involves importing preoperative CT scan data into an image guidance device. During surgery, this device uses technology to track the positions of surgical instruments and projects this information onto the preoperative CT images. This process enhances situational awareness for the surgeon. This is particularly useful when performing DRAF procedures.

11. **What are the different types of frontal sinus surgery/Draf procedures (Table 3.1)?**

3.2   Septoplasty

Indications for surgery [2]:

- Deviated nasal septum causing significant nasal obstruction
- Septal deviation contributing to obstructive sleep apnoea
- Septal perforations causing symptoms or requiring repair
- Epistaxis

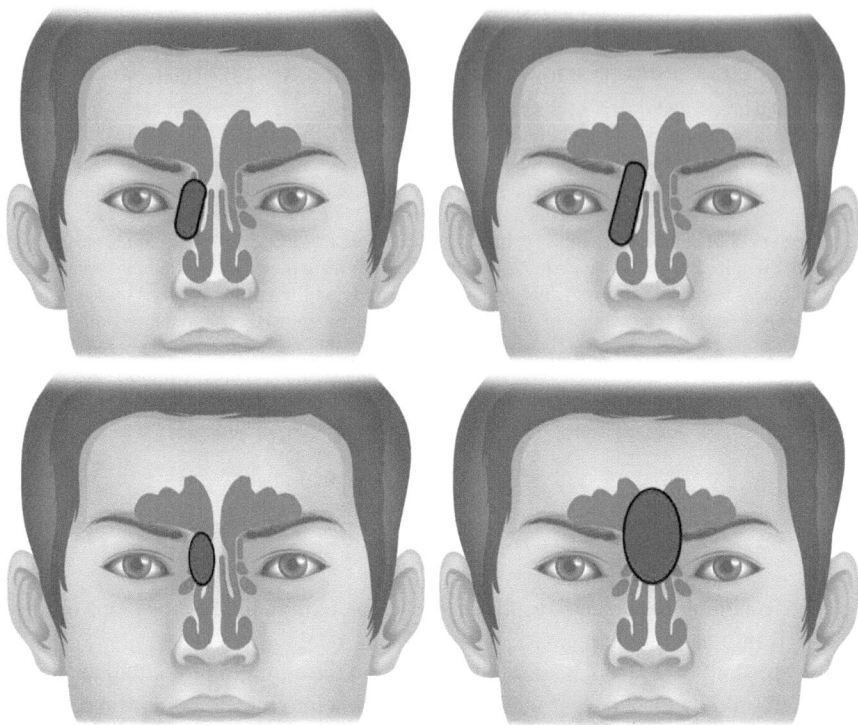

Fig. 3.2 Draf procedures visualized (Draf I, IIA, IIB, III). (Illustrated by Vikum Liyanaarachchi)

- As an adjunct to other nasal or sinus surgeries (e.g. chronic sinusitis, rhinoplasty, endoscopic sinus, and skull base surgeries)

Specific risks involved with the surgery [2]:

- Bleeding
- Infection
- Septal haematoma
- Recurrence of septal deviation
- Septal perforation (1–2%)
- Persistent or worsening nasal obstruction
- Change in nasal shape or appearance, including saddle nose deformity
- Olfactory disturbance or loss
- Adhesions or synechiae formation
- Septal cartilage necrosis (rare)

Preoperative Planning:

1. **Patient assessment**: Evaluate the patient's nasal structure, including both external and internal nasal examination, to determine the extent of septal deviation and its impact on nasal airflow. Assess for function, including the external and internal nasal valves, misting on metal speculum, and Cottle manoeuvre (gently pulling the ala/lateral wall of the nose laterally to assess the effect on breathing). Assess the patient's mental ability to cope with surgery and possible complications.

Surgical Steps:

1. General anaesthesia is used. Total intravenous anaesthesia (TIVA) is preferred for reducing intraoperative/post-operative bleeding. Prepare the nasal cavity with topical decongestants to reduce mucosal bleeding.
2. Administer local anaesthesia with a vasoconstrictor, e.g. 2% lidocaine with 1:80,000 adrenaline (Lignospan©).
3. The patient should be positioned supine on the operating table with their head elevated at about 15°–30°. This head-up position helps reduce venous pressure and minimize bleeding. The patient's head should be stabilized with a headrest, and the surgeon should ensure proper alignment to provide optimal access to the nasal structures.
4. Perform a hemitransfixion or Killian incision on one side of the caudal septum (usually left) to access the septal cartilage and bone (Fig. 3.3).
5. Carefully elevate the mucoperichondrial and mucoperiosteum using Iris scissors or Freer elevator to create a subperichondrial/subperiosteal pocket while

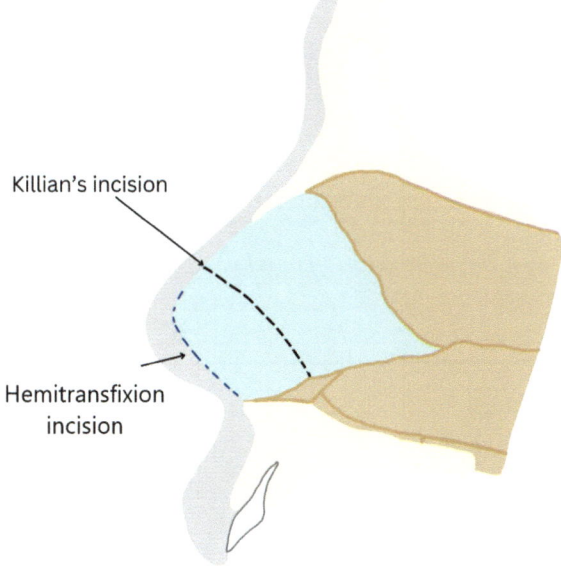

Fig. 3.3 Showing Killian's and hemitransfixion incision for septoplasty. (Illustrated by Vikum Liyanaarachchi)

preserving the mucosal integrity (avoiding tears). The septal cartilage has a bluish tinge and should be a bloodless plane. You may choose to elevate both mucoperichondrial flaps.
6. A posterior chondrotomy is performed by making an incision in the posterior cartilaginous part of the septum to separate it from the underlying bony structures, specifically the vomer and the perpendicular plate of the ethmoid bone.
7. Identify areas of cartilage and bone contributing to the deviation. Take care not to disrupt the keystone area (superiorly where the septum meets the nasal bones) and preserve the L-strut, which is crucial for maintaining nasal structure as seen in Fig. 3.4.
8. Remove or reshape deviated portions of the septal cartilage and perpendicular plate of the ethmoid bone, and vomer, using a Freer elevator, septal scissors, a scalpel, or a chisel. The goal is to maintain as much septal support as possible, to reduce the risk of saddle nose deformity. Consider the L-strut whenever removing cartilage (Fig. 3.4).
9. Realign the septum to the midline using sutures or splints if necessary. Additional techniques, such as cartilage grafts or spreader grafts, may be employed to straighten the septum and improve nasal support. A septal anchor/

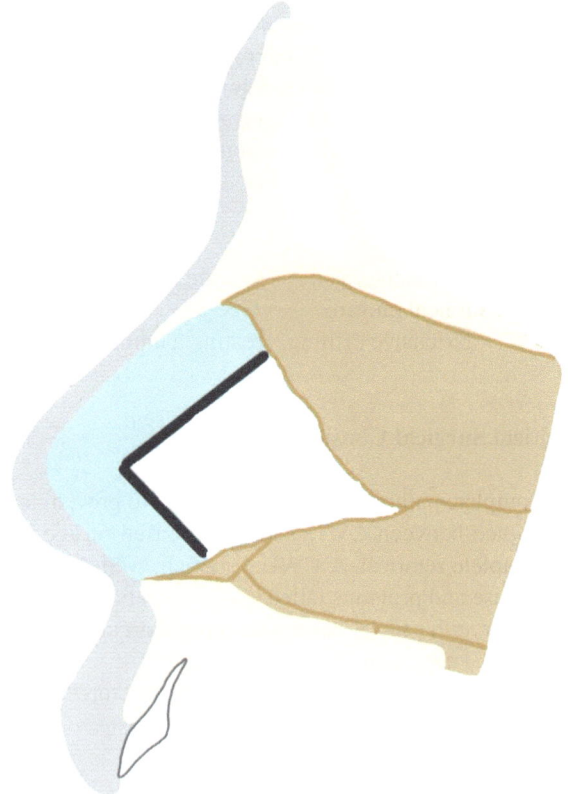

Fig. 3.4 L-strut shown in caudal cartilage (light blue). (Illustrated by Vikum Liyanaarachchi)

fixation suture can be placed from the inferior caudal septum into the anterior nasal spine.
10. It is good practice to crush the cartilage that has been removed, and place it back in the septum. This is known as cartilage recycling.
11. Reapproximate the mucosal flaps with absorbable sutures, to reduce the risk of haematoma formation. Place a soft nasal packing or septal splints to support the septum and reduce bleeding if required.

Post-operative Care:

- **Packing removal**: Unless soluble packing is used, remove the nasal packing/splint in clinic 1–2 weeks post-op to ensure proper healing.
- **Follow-up**: Schedule post-operative visits to monitor the healing process and address any complications such as infection or persistent deviation.

Complication Management:

- **Septal haematoma**: Monitor for swelling or discoloration of the septum post-operatively. If a haematoma is suspected, prompt intervention is required to evacuate the clot to prevent cartilage damage or infection.
- **Adhesions**: Prevent adhesions by ensuring precise mucosal approximation during closure and consider using septal splints. A visit within the first 3 weeks will allow for blunt division of adhesions forming between the septum and turbinate/s.
- **Nasal obstruction**: Re-evaluate the patient for persistent nasal obstruction, which may indicate residual or recurrent septal deviation, turbinate hypertrophy, or other intranasal pathology requiring further intervention.

Important points to note during the surgery:

- Preserve sufficient cartilage and bone framework to maintain septal support and prevent post-operative collapse.
- Minimize injury to the mucosal layers to reduce the risk of septal haematoma, perforation, or adhesions.
- Use atraumatic techniques and careful dissection to avoid injury to surrounding structures.
- Ensure adequate straightening of the septum to improve nasal airflow.

Questions a consultant might ask a trainee about the operation:

1. **What are the key anatomical landmarks to identify during septoplasty?**
    Key anatomical landmarks include the septal cartilage, perpendicular plate of the ethmoid bone, vomer bone, maxillary crest, and mucoperichondrial and mucoperiosteal layers.
2. **How do you minimize the risk of septal perforation during septoplasty?**

If you have a tear in the mucoperichondrial flap raised bilaterally in a similar position (i.e. both anterior), then this may compromise the blood supply to the septal cartilage causing a perforation to develop. To minimize the risk of septal perforation, ensure adequate elevation of the mucoperichondrial and mucoperiosteal flaps, avoid excessive force during dissection, and preserve a sufficient cartilage and bone framework to maintain septal support.

3. **What factors may contribute to post-operative nasal obstruction after septoplasty, and how can they be prevented?**

   Factors that may contribute to post-operative nasal obstruction include persistent and recurrent septal deviation, post-operative oedema, adhesions, or turbinate hypertrophy. To prevent post-operative nasal obstruction, ensure adequate straightening of the septum, minimize mucosal injury, and consider addressing other contributing factors such as turbinate hypertrophy during the surgery. Check for and divide adhesions during the post-op visit.

4. **How do you manage a septal haematoma after septoplasty?**

   In the case of a septal haematoma, promptly drain the haematoma, remove any clots, irrigate the cavity, and ensure adequate haemostasis. Repack the nasal cavity, consider using bilateral splints, and prescribe antibiotics to prevent infection.

5. **What are some potential complications of an untreated septal haematoma, and why is it important to address them promptly?**

   Potential complications of an untreated septal haematoma include septal perforation, infection, cartilage necrosis, and saddle nose deformity. Promptly addressing a septal haematoma is important to prevent these complications, especially infection which may spread intracranially (dangerous area of the face), and to preserve the structural integrity of the nasal septum and ensure optimal post-operative outcomes.

6. **What are the structures that form the nasal septum?**

   The nasal septum is formed by several key structures, including the quadrangular cartilage, the perpendicular plate of the ethmoid bone, the vomer, the maxillary crest, and the palatine crest.

7. **How are post-operative septal perforations managed?**

   Management of post-operative septal perforations depends on the severity of symptoms. If the perforation is asymptomatic, no intervention is required, but the patient should be advised on what symptoms to watch for. For mild symptoms such as crusting or bleeding, conservative medical management is recommended, including nasal douching, Vaseline, Nasogel©, or Naseptin© cream. If the symptoms affect the quality of life or cause a saddle nose deformity, surgical management should be considered. Surgical options include using a prosthesis (septal button) or employing local flaps, such as a bi-pedicled advancement flap, an anterior ethmoidal artery septal flap, a facial artery myomucosal (FAMM) flap, or a rotational mucosal flap with an acellular dermal interposition graft.

8. **What is the small spherical structure in the nasal septum?**

   The small spherical structure in the nasal septum is Jacobson's organ or the vomeronasal organ. It is located in the anterior third of the nasal septum, above the hard palate. In animals, it is thought to be responsible for the secretion of pheromones, though its function in humans remains unclear. This organ is connected to the cranial nerve terminalis, which links to the accessory olfactory bulb, sending neurons to the hypothalamus.

3.3 Turbinectomy/Turbinoplasty

Indications for surgery [3]:

- Chronic nasal obstruction due to inferior turbinate hypertrophy, unresponsive to medical treatment
- Allergic rhinitis with significant turbinate hypertrophy, unresponsive to medical treatment
- Concha bullosa causing nasal obstruction or recurrent sinusitis
- As an adjunct to other nasal or sinus surgeries (e.g. septoplasty, endoscopic sinus surgery)

Specific risks involved with the surgery [3]:

- Bleeding
- Infection
- Dryness or crusting of the nasal mucosa
- Olfactory disturbance or loss
- Empty nose syndrome
- Adhesions or synechiae formation
- Persistent or worsening nasal obstruction

Steps of the surgery:

1. General anaesthesia is used. Total intravenous anaesthesia (TIVA) is preferred for reducing intraoperative/post-operative bleeding. Prepare the nasal cavity with topical decongestants to reduce mucosal bleeding.
2. Administer local anaesthesia with a vasoconstrictor, e.g. 2% lidocaine with 1:80,000 adrenaline (Lignospan©).
3. The patient should be positioned supine on the operating table with their head elevated at about 15°–30°. This head-up position helps reduce venous pressure and minimize bleeding. The patient's head should be stabilized with a headrest, and the surgeon should ensure proper alignment to provide optimal access to the nasal structures.
4. Employ a submucosal approach, making a conservative incision along the anterior edge of the inferior turbinate to preserve mucosal tissue and avoid atrophic rhinitis.

5. **Submucosal dissection**: Elevate the mucosal layer from the underlying turbinate bone using blunt dissection to create a submucosal tunnel, sparing the overlying ciliated epithelium.
6. **Soft tissue reduction**: Utilize radiofrequency ablation, laser, or a microdebrider to reduce the volume of the hypertrophic turbinates, taking care to avoid thermal injury to the surrounding tissues.
7. **Bone resection**: If indicated, out fracture the turbinate bone gently, and remove the bony portion using bone-cutting forceps or a microdebrider with a bone shaver attachment, ensuring that the lateral nasal wall and nasal septum are not compromised.
8. **Haemostasis**: Achieve haemostasis with electrocautery. Topical application of haemostatic agents may also be used such as adrenaline.
9. **Closure**: Typically, no suturing is required as the mucosal flaps will adhere naturally. A dissolvable packing may be placed to support the tissue and prevent synechiae formation.

Important points to note during the surgery:

- Preserve sufficient turbinate tissue to maintain normal nasal function and prevent complications such as dryness or empty nose syndrome.
- Minimize injury to the surrounding mucosa to reduce the risk of adhesions, synechiae, or scarring.
- Use atraumatic techniques and careful dissection to avoid injury to surrounding structures.
- Ensure adequate improvement of the nasal airflow.

Questions a consultant might ask a trainee about the operation:

1. **What is the role of the turbinates in nasal physiology, and why is it important to preserve their function?**
    The turbinates play a crucial role in nasal physiology by humidifying, warming, and filtering the inspired air, as well as regulating nasal resistance and airflow [3]. Preserving their function helps maintain a healthy nasal environment and prevents complications such as dryness, crusting, or empty nose syndrome.
2. **What are some different techniques for performing turbinectomy/turbinoplasty, and how do you choose the appropriate technique for a specific patient?**
    Techniques for turbinectomy/turbinoplasty (Fig. 3.5) include submucosal resection, radiofrequency ablation, laser-assisted turbinoplasty, microdebrider-assisted turbinoplasty, linear submucosal cautery (using Abbey needle), and out fracture or lateralization. The choice of technique depends on the patient's specific anatomy, the severity of the hypertrophy, and the surgeon's experience and preference.
3. **What factors may contribute to persistent or worsening nasal obstruction after turbinectomy/turbinoplasty, and how can they be prevented?**

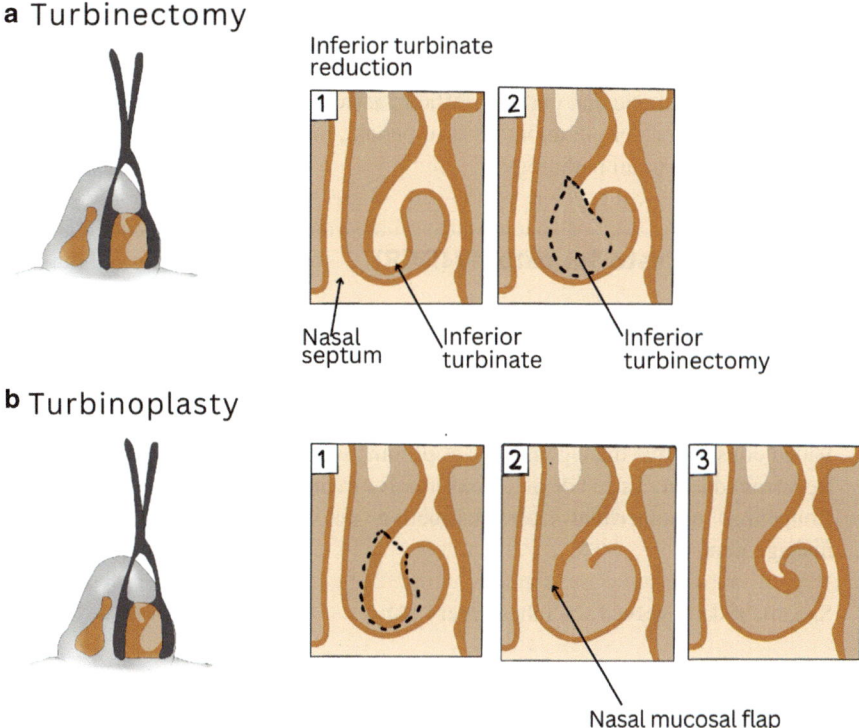

Fig. 3.5 Showing turbinectomy (**a**) and turbinoplasty (**b**). (Illustrated by Vikum Liyanaarachchi)

Factors that may contribute to persistent or worsening nasal obstruction include inadequate turbinate reduction, post-operative oedema, adhesions, or other untreated anatomical abnormalities (e.g. septal deviation). To prevent these issues, ensure adequate improvement of the nasal airflow during the surgery, minimize mucosal injury, and consider addressing other contributing factors such as septal deviation or addressing other nasal anatomical issues during the surgery. Note the possibility of a paradoxical persistent sense of nasal obstruction as part of empty nose syndrome, where the nasal airway is patent.

4. **What is empty nose syndrome, and how can it be prevented during turbinectomy/turbinoplasty?**

   Empty nose syndrome is a rare complication characterized by dryness, crusting, and a paradoxical sensation of nasal congestion, despite the wide-open nasal passages. It is a rare complication that may lead to significant psychological symptoms including anxiety, depression, and suicidal thoughts. It is usually associated with overly aggressive turbinectomy, which impairs normal nasal physiology. To prevent empty nose syndrome, preserve sufficient turbinate tissue during the surgery, use conservative techniques, and focus on maintaining normal nasal function.

5. **What is the nasal cycle?**

The nasal cycle refers to the cycles of alternating congestion and decongestion of the two nasal cavities, including the turbinate mucosa. These cycles can last from minutes to hours throughout the day and are related to the balance between sympathetic and parasympathetic activity. The nasal cycle is a subconscious process present in about 80% of people, but it becomes more noticeable in patients with nasal pathology.

3.4 Dacryocystorhinostomy (DCR)

Indications for surgery [4]:

- Nasolacrimal duct obstruction causing epiphora (excessive tearing) or dacryocystitis (infection of the lacrimal sac)
- Failed conservative management (e.g. probing, intubation, or irrigation)
- Recurrent dacryocystitis despite conservative treatment
- Congenital nasolacrimal duct obstruction not resolving with conservative management

Specific risks involved with the surgery [4]:

- Bleeding
- Infection
- Scarring or stenosis at the anastomosis site
- Failure to resolve epiphora or dacryocystitis
- Injury to the medial canthal tendon
- Orbital injury or haematoma
- Unmasking of underlying dry eye syndrome
- Cerebrospinal fluid (CSF) leak (rare)

Steps of the surgery:

1. General anaesthesia is used. Total intravenous anaesthesia (TIVA) is preferred for reducing intraoperative/post-operative bleeding. Prepare the nasal cavity with topical decongestants to reduce mucosal bleeding.
2. Administer local anaesthesia with a vasoconstrictor, e.g. 2% lidocaine with 1:80,000 adrenaline (Lignospan©).
3. The patient should be positioned supine on the operating table with their head elevated at about 15°–30°. This head-up position helps reduce venous pressure and minimize bleeding. The patient's head should be stabilized with a headrest, and the surgeon should ensure proper alignment to provide optimal access to the nasal structures.
4. Insert a 0° or 30° endoscope into the nasal cavity, illuminating the lateral nasal wall to identify the lacrimal sac fossa, which lies anterior and inferior to the middle turbinate.

5. Raise a mucoperiosteal flap.
6. **Osteotomy**: Carefully create an osteotomy over the lacrimal sac fossa using a high-speed drill or Kerrison rongeurs, taking care to preserve the integrity of the lacrimal sac.
7. **Sac incision**: Open the lacrimal sac vertically to expose the medial and lateral flaps, ensuring that the incision is large enough to allow for adequate drainage.
8. **Flap anastomosis**: Suture the lacrimal sac flaps to the lateral nasal mucosa to create a direct communication between the lacrimal sac and the nasal cavity, which facilitates tear drainage.
9. **Stenting**: Place a silicone stent through the new ostium into the lacrimal drainage system to maintain patency, typically left in place for several weeks to months. See Fig. 3.6.
10. **Closure**: The mucoperiosteal flap is repositioned without suturing, and the nose is typically not packed unless significant bleeding is encountered.

Important points to note during the surgery:

- Proper patient selection and preoperative assessment (e.g. dacryocystography, nasal endoscopy) to identify the cause of the obstruction and plan the surgical approach.
- Minimize injury to surrounding structures, such as the medial canthal tendon or orbital contents.
- Ensure adequate exposure of the lacrimal sac and nasal mucosa for a successful anastomosis.
- Properly secure and position the stent (if used) to maintain patency and avoid complications.

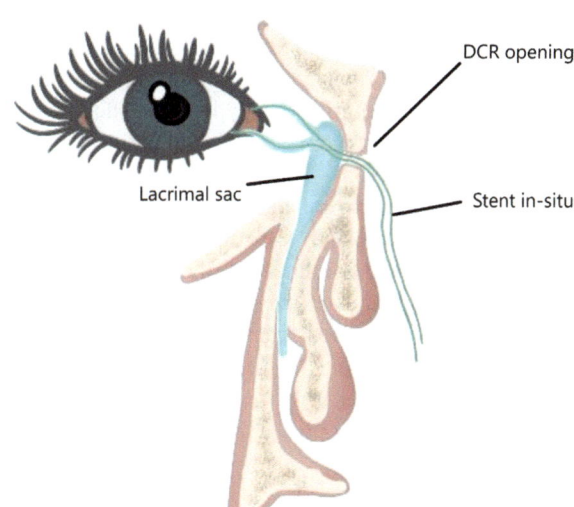

Fig. 3.6 DCR performed and stent placed in situ. (Illustrated by Vikum Liyanaarachchi)

Questions a consultant might ask a trainee about the operation:

1. **What are the key anatomical landmarks to identify during DCR?**
   Key anatomical landmarks include the medial canthal tendon, anterior aspect of the middle turbinate, lacrimal sac fossa, lacrimal sac, nasal mucosa, and nasolacrimal duct [4].
2. **What are the main differences between external and endoscopic DCR, and how do you choose the appropriate approach for a specific patient?**
   External DCR involves a skin incision and dissection to expose the lacrimal sac, while endoscopic DCR is performed entirely through the nasal cavity using an endoscope. The choice of approach depends on the patient's specific anatomy, the cause of the obstruction, the surgeon's experience and preference, and the availability of appropriate equipment.
3. **How do you minimize the risk of scarring or stenosis at the anastomosis site during DCR?**
   To minimize the risk of scarring or stenosis, ensure adequate exposure and dissection of the lacrimal sac and nasal mucosa, create a sufficiently large osteotomy, and consider the placement of a temporary stent to maintain patency.
4. **What factors may contribute to the failure of DCR, and how can they be prevented or addressed?**
   Factors that may contribute to the failure of DCR include inadequate osteotomy size, scarring or stenosis at the anastomosis site, improper stent placement, or other unaddressed anatomical abnormalities (e.g. nasal polyps or sinusitis). To prevent or address these issues, ensure adequate exposure and dissection, create a sufficiently large osteotomy, properly secure and position the stent (if used), and address any other contributing factors during the surgery [4].
5. **How do you manage a patient with persistent epiphora or dacryocystitis after DCR?**
   In cases of persistent epiphora or dacryocystitis after DCR, re-evaluate the patient to determine the cause of the failure. Consider additional imaging, such as dacryocystography, to assess the anastomosis and identify any remaining obstruction. Depending on the findings, additional interventions such as revision DCR, balloon dacryoplasty, or nasolacrimal duct stenting may be necessary to address the problem.
6. **Describe the anatomical drainage of the lacrimal apparatus?**
   The lacrimal gland is in the anterior orbit within the lacrimal fossa of the frontal bone. Tears produced by the gland pass through the puncta of the superior lacrimal canaliculus in the upper eyelid and the inferior lacrimal canaliculus in the lower eyelid. These canaliculi usually join to form a common canaliculus, which drains tears into the lacrimal sac. From the lacrimal sac, tears flow through the nasolacrimal duct, which ends in the inferior meatus by the valve of Hasner.
7. **How could you identify clinically the level of obstruction in the lacrimal apparatus?**
   The modified Jones test is used to identify the level of obstruction:

First part: A drop of fluorescein is placed in the conjunctiva. After 5 min, the nose is examined for the presence of dye. If no dye is present, an obstruction is indicated, prompting the second part of the test.

Second part: A cannula is inserted into the lacrimal sac, which is then flushed with saline. If no fluorescein is observed, the dye is obstructed in the upper (canalicular) portion of the system. If dye is present, the obstruction is in the lower (sac or duct) portion.

Additionally, the regurgitation test can be performed by applying pressure over the lacrimal sac with an index finger or thumb and observing the puncta. In cases of nasolacrimal duct obstruction, regurgitation occurs through the punctum.

3.5 Endoscopic Skull Base Surgery

Indications for surgery [5]:

- Benign or malignant skull base tumours (e.g. pituitary adenomas, craniopharyngiomas, chordomas, meningiomas, SCC), applicable to where equivalent results to open surgery have been achieved with endoscopic surgery
- Cerebrospinal fluid (CSF) leaks
- Inflammatory or infectious conditions (e.g. mucoceles, fungal sinusitis)
- Traumatic injuries or fractures involving the skull base

Specific risks involved with the surgery [5]:

- Bleeding
- Infection
- CSF leak or meningitis
- Injury to the brain, nerves, or blood vessels
- Loss of olfactory, visual, or other neurological function
- Endocrine dysfunction (e.g. diabetes insipidus, hypopituitarism)
- Post-operative scarring or adhesions
- Incomplete resection of tumour
- Need to convert to conventional surgical approach
- Risk of seizures including being unable to drive for 6 months (when temporal lobe retraction is needed)

Various approaches to endoscopic skull base surgery:

1. Transnasal approach (endoscopic endonasal approach, EEA):
   - Access through the nasal cavity and paranasal sinuses
   - Indicated for lesions in the anterior and central skull base, such as pituitary adenomas, craniopharyngiomas, and olfactory groove meningiomas
2. Transethmoidal approach:
   - Access through the ethmoid sinus

- Indicated for lesions in the ethmoid sinus, planum sphenoidale, and cribriform plate region, such as olfactory groove meningiomas and anterior skull base encephaloceles
3. Transsphenoidal approach:
   - Access through the sphenoid sinus
   - Indicated for lesions in the sellar and parasellar regions, such as pituitary adenomas, Rathke's cleft cysts, and craniopharyngiomas
4. Transpterygoid approach:
   - Access through the maxillary and sphenopalatine foramina
   - Indicated for lesions in the lateral skull base, such as juvenile angiofibroma, infratemporal fossa tumours, and petrous apex lesions
5. Transorbital approach:
   - Access through the orbit or the superior and inferior orbital fissures
   - Indicated for lesions in the orbital apex, cavernous sinus, and middle fossa, such as orbital tumours, cavernous sinus meningiomas, and trigeminal schwannomas

Important points to note during the surgery:

- Proper patient selection and preoperative assessment, including imaging (e.g. CT, MRI) and endoscopic evaluation, to determine the appropriate surgical approach
- A thorough understanding of the complex skull base anatomy and potential variations in individual patients
- Minimized injury to surrounding structures, such as the brain, nerves, and blood vessels
- Use of advanced endoscopic equipment and surgical instruments for precise dissection and visualization
- Collaboration with a multidisciplinary team, including neurosurgeons, otolaryngologists, and anaesthesiologists, to optimize patient outcomes
- Surgical skill set to include expert-level skills in sinus surgery, with the ability to perform more extensive procedures as may be required to effect excision

Endoscopic Endonasal Transsphenoidal Approach for Pituitary Adenomas
Steps of the surgery:

1. Patient positioning: Place the patient in a supine position with the head slightly extended and secured in a three-pin head holder.
2. Anaesthesia and monitoring: Administer general anaesthesia with endotracheal intubation. Perform continuous neurophysiological monitoring, such as visual evoked potentials (VEPs) and electroencephalography (EEG), to assess the function of the optic nerves and brain throughout the surgery.
3. Nasal decongestion and preparation: Apply topical vasoconstrictors (e.g. oxymetazoline or phenylephrine) to the nasal mucosa to reduce bleeding and facilitate exposure.

4. Endoscope insertion: Introduce a 0°, 4 mm endoscope into one nostril, typically the right nostril for a right-handed surgeon.
5. Nasal septum elevation: Identify the middle turbinate, and elevate the nasal septal mucosa bilaterally, preserving the mucoperiosteum. This step is optional and depends on the surgeon's preference and the specific anatomy of the patient.
6. Sphenoidotomy: Identify the sphenoid ostium in the sphenoethmoidal recess, and perform a wide sphenoidotomy, removing the posterior part of the nasal septum and the rostrum of the sphenoid bone to expose the sphenoid sinus.
7. Sphenoid sinus exploration: Remove any sphenoid sinus septations, and identify the sella turcica, carotid protuberances, and opticocarotid recesses.
8. Sellar floor opening: Create a small opening in the sellar floor using a high-speed drill or other appropriate instruments, taking care not to damage the underlying dura mater.
9. Dura mater incision: Perform a cruciate incision on the dura mater, and carefully retract it to expose the pituitary adenoma.
10. Tumour removal: Using microsurgical instruments, such as curettes, suction devices, and pituitary rongeurs, perform a systematic and piecemeal resection of the pituitary adenoma. Use gentle traction and internal debulking to preserve the surrounding pituitary gland and avoid injury to the adjacent structures, such as the cavernous sinus, optic chiasm, and carotid arteries.
11. Haemostasis and reconstruction: Achieve haemostasis using bipolar electrocautery, haemostatic agents, or Surgicel. If a CSF leak is encountered or if there is a high risk of post-operative CSF leak, perform multi-layered reconstruction using various materials, such as autologous fat grafts, fascia lata, or synthetic dural substitutes. In some cases, additional support with a vascularized nasoseptal flap may be necessary.
12. Nasal packing and closure: Place a nasal pack, such as Merocel or Floseal, to provide gentle compression and minimize post-operative bleeding. The nasal pack is usually removed 1–2 days after surgery.
13. Post-operative care: Monitor the patient closely for any signs of complications, such as CSF leak, meningitis, or visual disturbances. Assess the patient's endocrine function, and provide appropriate hormone replacement therapy, if necessary. Perform post-operative imaging (e.g. MRI) to evaluate the extent of tumour resection and guide further management, such as adjuvant radiotherapy or additional surgery, if needed.

Important points to note during the surgery:

- Maintain a clear surgical field with good visualization throughout the procedure. Use a 30° endoscope for angled views, if necessary. Frequent irrigation and suction may be needed to clear blood and debris.
- Be aware of the potential for anatomical variations, such as Onodi cells, which can increase the risk of injury to the optic nerve or carotid artery. Adjust the surgical approach accordingly based on the individual patient's anatomy.

- Minimize injury to the normal pituitary gland and surrounding structures, such as the optic chiasm, cavernous sinus, and carotid arteries. Avoid excessive traction, sharp dissection, or bipolar cautery near these structures.
- If a CSF leak is encountered or anticipated, use a multi-layered reconstruction technique and consider lumbar drainage to reduce the risk of post-operative CSF leak and meningitis.

Questions a consultant might ask a trainee about the operation:

1. **How do you determine the most appropriate endoscopic approach for a specific skull base lesion? What are the key anatomical landmarks to identify during these approaches?**

    The choice of approach depends on the lesion's location, size, and extent, as well as the patient's anatomy and the surgeon's experience. Here are the main approaches and their key landmarks:

    Transnasal approach (endoscopic endonasal approach, EEA): Access through the nasal cavity and paranasal sinuses. Indicated for lesions in the anterior and central skull base, such as pituitary adenomas, craniopharyngiomas, and olfactory groove meningiomas. Key landmarks: middle turbinate, sphenoid ostium, sella turcica, carotid protuberances, opticocarotid recesses, and dura mater.

    Transethmoidal approach: Access through the ethmoid sinus. Indicated for lesions in the ethmoid sinus, planum sphenoidale, and cribriform plate region, such as olfactory groove meningiomas and anterior skull base encephaloceles. Key landmarks: ethmoid sinuses and cribriform plate.

    Transsphenoidal approach: Access through the sphenoid sinus. Indicated for lesions in the sellar and parasellar regions, such as pituitary adenomas, Rathke's cleft cysts, and craniopharyngiomas. Key landmarks: sphenoid sinus, sella turcica, carotid arteries, and optic nerves.

    Transpterygoid approach: Access through the maxillary and sphenopalatine foramina. Indicated for lesions in the lateral skull base, such as juvenile angiofibromas, infratemporal fossa tumours, and petrous apex lesions. Key landmarks: maxillary sinus and pterygopalatine fossa.

    Transorbital approach: Access through the orbit or the superior and inferior orbital fissures. Indicated for lesions in the orbital apex, cavernous sinus, and middle fossa, such as orbital tumours, cavernous sinus meningiomas, and trigeminal schwannomas. Key landmarks: orbital apex and cavernous sinus.

    Preoperative imaging (CT/MRI) and endoscopic evaluation help in choosing the best approach based on the lesion's characteristics and critical surrounding structures.

2. **How do you minimize the risk of post-operative complications such as CSF leak, meningitis, or injury to critical structures like the optic nerve or carotid artery during endoscopic skull base surgery?**

    To minimize complications:
    - Use precise dissection techniques, and handle tissues carefully.
    - Preserve critical structures such as nerves and blood vessels.

- Employ gentle dissection techniques, avoiding excessive traction or sharp dissection near the optic nerve or carotid artery, and be aware of anatomical variations like Onodi cells.
- For CSF leaks, use a multi-layered closure technique with autologous fascia lata, fat grafts, or synthetic dural substitutes, and consider post-operative lumbar drainage.

3. **How can you identify and manage a CSF leakage site intraoperatively? What post-operative care is recommended following a CSF leak?**

    To identify a CSF leak intraoperatively:
    - Ask the anaesthetist to perform the Valsalva manoeuvre and lower the head of the bed.
    - Use intrathecal fluorescein (off-label in the UK) to visualize the leak.
    - To manage a CSF leak:
    - For small defects, use the bath plug fat underlay technique (mushroom repair).
    - For larger defects, employ a multi-layer overlay technique with flaps such as the Hadad flap (naso-septal pedicled flap).
    - Post-operative care includes:
    - Bed rest with the head elevated 15°–30°.
    - Use laxatives to avoid straining.
    - Consider prophylactic antibiotics (controversial).
    - Use lumbar drainage and diuretics for high CSF pressure cases.

4. **What are the indications for considering an alternative approach for pituitary adenoma resection using the endoscopic endonasal transsphenoidal approach?**

    Consider alternative approaches, such as the transcranial or subcranial approach, for:
    - Large or giant pituitary adenomas with significant suprasellar or parasellar extension
    - Tumours invading the cavernous sinus
    - Tumours with significant involvement of the optic chiasm or nerves
    - Cases with previous transsphenoidal surgery where scar tissue or altered anatomy complicates the endonasal approach

5. **How do you manage intraoperative bleeding during endoscopic skull base surgery?**

    Managing intraoperative bleeding involves:
    - Identifying and controlling the source of bleeding quickly
    - Using haemostatic agents and bipolar cautery for minor bleeding
    - Employing packing or tamponade techniques for moderate bleeding
    - In cases of significant bleeding, temporarily halting the procedure to stabilize the patient, potentially involving interventional radiology for embolization, or converting to an open approach if necessary
    - Maintaining clear visualization with continuous irrigation and suction

3.6 Rhinoplasty

Indications for surgery [6]:

- Aesthetic improvement of the nose shape, size, or symmetry
- Correction of nasal deformities (e.g. dorsal hump, saddle nose, crooked nose)
- Improvement of nasal function (e.g. alleviating nasal obstruction with complex septal deformity, particularly if it involves the external or internal nasal valves)
- Repair of nasal trauma or previous surgery complications

Relative contraindications to surgery [6]:

- A mismatch between the patient expectations and the expected surgical outcome.
- Low psychological reserve, with the patient unable to mentally manage the potential change and possible complications.
- Concerns about body dysmorphic disorder (BDD)—high incidence in cosmetic rhinoplasty population.
- "SIMON" (single, immature, male, overexpecting, narcissistic) vs. "SYLVIA" (secure, young, listens, verbal, intelligent, attractive) is useful when defining the ideal patient, but not much help in individual cases.
- Surgeon's intuitive feeling of disliking the patient may be the only warning of BDD.

Specific risks involved with the surgery [6]:

- Bleeding
- Infection
- Anaesthesia complications
- Unsatisfactory cosmetic results
- Numbness of tip of nose and upper teeth
- Recurrence of septal deviation and adhesions leading to persistent nasal obstruction or difficulty breathing (risk often quoted as around 10%)
- Septal perforation or haematoma (risk often quoted as around 1%, which may lead to crusting, nosebleeds, and, in some cases, whistling noise while breathing through the nose)
- Asymmetry or irregularities
- Need for revision surgery (risk normally regarded as around 10%)
- Skin soft tissue contractures
- Skin necrosis (higher risk with revision surgery)
- Psychological distress

Preoperative planning: Evaluate the patient's nasal anatomy, skin thickness, and facial proportions. Discuss the patient's goals and expectations, and develop a surgical plan. The patient requires photographic imaging from eight different angles.

Steps of the surgery:

3 Rhinology

1. General anaesthesia is used. Total intravenous anaesthesia (TIVA) is preferred for reducing intraoperative/post-operative bleeding. Prepare the nasal cavity with topical decongestants to reduce mucosal bleeding.
2. Administer local anaesthesia with a vasoconstrictor, e.g. 2% lidocaine with 1:80,000 adrenaline (Lignospan©).
3. The patient should be positioned supine on the operating table with their head elevated at about 15°–30°. This head-up position helps reduce venous pressure and minimize bleeding. The patient's head should be stabilized with a headrest, and the surgeon should ensure proper alignment to provide optimal access to the nasal structures.

Open approach:

4. Perform a columellar incision (Fig. 3.7): using an inverted-V or stair-step pattern. Then proceed to make additional incisions inside the nostrils. These typically include marginal, intercartilaginous, and transfixion incisions.
    (a) Columellar incision: Begin with the inverted-V or stair-step incision across the columella. This allows for precise alignment during closure and minimizes visible scarring.

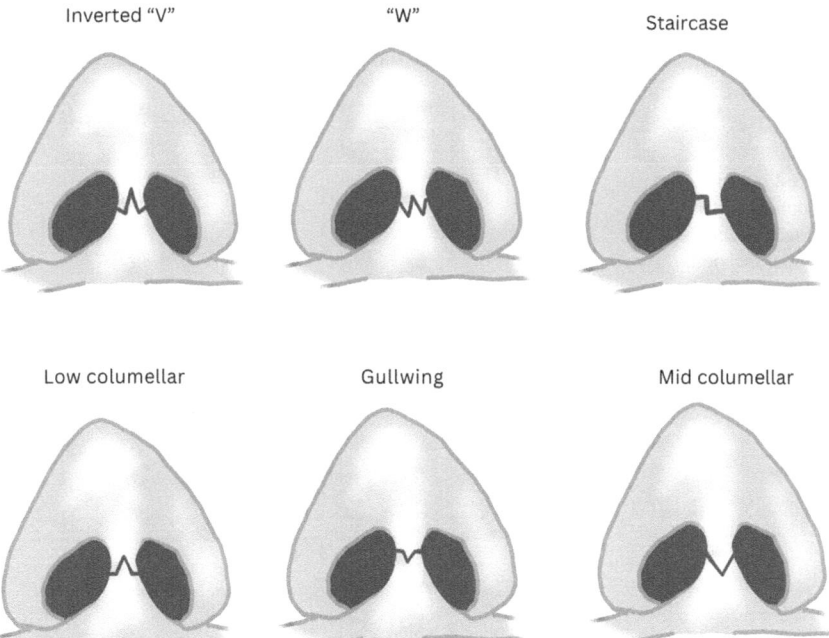

Fig. 3.7 Different incisions used in open-approach rhinoplasty. (Illustrated by Vikum Liyanaarachchi)

(b) Marginal incision: Make an incision along the lower edge of the alar cartilage, following the natural contour of the nostril. This provides access to the lower lateral cartilages, as seen in Fig. 3.8.
(c) Intercartilaginous incision: Make this incision between the upper and lower lateral cartilages. It allows access to the nasal tip and dorsum and helps in mobilizing the cartilages.
(d) Transfixion incision: Make this incision through the septum just behind the columella. It aids in accessing and straightening the nasal septum and provides additional exposure.

Closed approach:

Intercartilaginous incision (as above):

- Using fine scissors or a scalpel, gently dissect the skin and soft tissue from the underlying nasal framework through the intercartilaginous incision.
- Carefully lift the skin and soft tissue off the upper lateral cartilages and nasal dorsum. Use a combination of sharp dissection (with a scalpel) and blunt dissection (using an elevator or periosteal elevator) to separate the skin and soft tissue. This step should be done meticulously to maintain the integrity of the skin flap and avoid damage to underlying structures.

Marginal incision (if needed):

- If additional access is required, make a marginal incision along the lower edge of the alar cartilage.

Fig. 3.8 Open-approach rhinoplasty with inverted-V incision + marginal incision

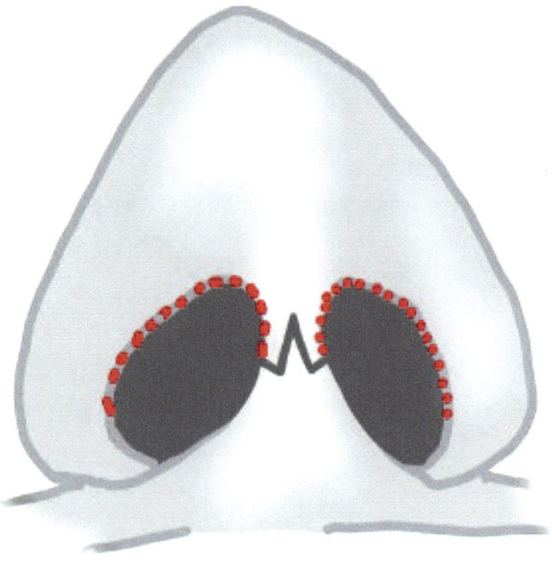

3 Rhinology

- Elevate the skin and soft tissue from the lower lateral cartilages, being careful to avoid excessive force to prevent tearing the skin flap. Use small retractors to hold the skin and provide a clear view of the cartilages.

Transfixion incision (if needed):

- If septal modification is necessary, make a transfixion incision through the septum just behind the columella.
- Carefully dissect along the septal cartilage, ensuring clear visualization and avoiding damage to the mucosal lining. This helps in straightening and modifying the septum if required.

5. Once these incisions are made, you can start the dissection process:
   (a) Using fine scissors or a scalpel, gently dissect the skin and soft tissue from the nasal framework. Begin at the columellar incision and extend the dissection upwards. Employ a combination of sharp dissection (with a scalpel) and blunt dissection to carefully separate the skin from the lower lateral cartilages. This step should be done meticulously to maintain the integrity of the skin flap and avoid damage to cartilage.
   (b) As you proceed, the goal is to expose the lower lateral cartilages. Carefully lift the skin and soft tissue over these cartilages, continuing the dissection laterally. During this process, avoid excessive force to prevent tearing the skin flap. Use small retractors to hold the skin and provide a clear view of the cartilages.
   (c) Once the lower lateral cartilages are adequately exposed, continue the dissection to reveal the upper lateral cartilages and nasal dorsum, if required.
6. Reshaping the nasal framework: Once the soft tissue is lifted off the bony and cartilaginous structures, perform the necessary modifications based on the patient's specific goals and anatomy. These modifications may include:
   Cartilage reshaping:
- Remove or reshape the cartilage as needed to achieve the desired contour.
- Use suture techniques, such as dome-binding sutures, for tip refinement.
- Consider using grafts for additional support and structure. For example, a spreader graft can be useful for internal nasal valve collapse, while alar batten grafts or columellar strut grafts can support the nasal structure and improve nasal airflow.
   Nasal hump reduction:
- Reduce the nasal hump using a rasp or osteotome, ensuring a smooth and natural contour.
   Tip refinement:
- Trim or reshape the lower lateral cartilages to refine the nasal tip. Techniques such as cephalic trim or dome-binding sutures can enhance tip definition and projection.

7. Osteotomies: If necessary, perform medial and/or lateral osteotomies to narrow the nasal bones and close the open roof after hump reduction.
   Medial osteotomies:
   - Perform medial osteotomies if necessary to narrow the nasal bones and close the open roof created after hump reduction. Use a guarded osteotome to make precise cuts along the medial aspect of the nasal bones.
   Lateral osteotomies:
   - Perform lateral osteotomies to further narrow the nasal bridge and bring the nasal bones closer together. This helps achieve a more refined nasal profile. Use a guarded osteotome to make controlled cuts along the lateral aspect of the nasal bones, ensuring that the cuts are symmetric and precise.
8. Septoplasty and/or turbinoplasty (if needed): If the patient has a deviated septum or enlarged turbinates causing nasal obstruction, correct these issues during the surgery.
9. Re-draping and closure: Carefully re-drape the skin and soft tissue over the modified nasal framework, ensuring a smooth contour. Close the incisions with fine sutures. In the case of an open approach, close the columellar incision with either continuous or interrupted sutures.
10. External nasal splint and internal nasal packing: Apply an external nasal splint to maintain the new shape and provide support during the initial healing phase. If necessary, place internal nasal packing to control bleeding and maintain the septal position.

    Important points to note during the surgery:

- Preserve the structural integrity of the nose while making modifications to the cartilage and bone.
- Use careful dissection techniques to minimize tissue trauma and bleeding.
- Ensure that the patient's breathing function is preserved or improved during the surgery.
- Closely monitor the patient's intraoperative and post-operative condition to detect any complications early.

Questions a consultant might ask a trainee about the operation:

1. **What are the advantages and disadvantages of the open versus closed rhinoplasty approach?**

   Open approach advantages include better visualization, easier access to nasal structures, and precise graft placement. Disadvantages include a visible columellar scar, increased swelling, and a longer recovery period. Closed approach advantages include no visible external scars, reduced swelling, and a shorter recovery period. Disadvantages include limited visualization and more challenging access to nasal structures.

2. **What are some common graft materials used in rhinoplasty, and what are their indications?**

Common graft materials include autologous cartilage (septal, auricular, or costal), which is preferred due to its biocompatibility and low risk of complications. Grafts can be used for various purposes, such as spreader grafts to improve the internal nasal valve, alar batten grafts to support the lateral nasal wall, and columellar strut grafts to provide tip support and projection.

3. **How do you manage a patient who is dissatisfied with their rhinoplasty results?**

    First, listen carefully to the patient's concerns and assess the surgical outcome objectively. If the concern is related to post-operative swelling, advise the patient to wait until the swelling has resolved, which may take several months. If the concern is related to a surgical issue or complication, discuss the possibility of revision surgery, which should be performed after an appropriate healing period (usually at least 1 year after the initial surgery).

4. **What are the major tip support mechanisms?**
    - The shape, size, and strength of the lower lateral cartilage
    - The attachment of the medial crural footplate to the caudal septum
    - The scroll area between the lower lateral cartilage and upper lateral cartilage [6]

5. **What are the minor tip support mechanisms:**
    - Anterior nasal spine
    - Lateral sesamoid cartilages
    - Interdomal ligaments
    - Caudal membranous septum
    - Dorsal septum
    - Skin and soft tissue envelope overlying the nasal tip [6]

6. **What is Anderson's tripod concept?**

    Anderson's tripod concept explains that the two lower lateral cartilages form a functional tripod providing tip support. The right and left lateral crura act as two legs of the tripod, and the conjoined medial crura function as the third leg. This concept helps predict how changes to these structures affect tip position.

7. **What are the boundaries of the external nasal valve and the internal nasal valve?**

    External nasal valve:
    - Alar cartilage
    - Caudal septum and columella
    - Nasal sill
    - Internal nasal valve (narrowest part of the nasal cavity):
    - Caudal edge of upper lateral cartilage
    - Dorsal septum
    - Anterior edge of inferior turbinate

8. **What are the angles required for photography pre- and post-rhinoplasty?**

    For pre- and post-rhinoplasty photography, the patient should have the following views:
    - Frontal view
    - Right and left lateral views
    - Right and left three-quarters oblique views

- Basal view
- Smiling view
- "Bird's-eye" frontal view with the chin tucked at 45°

3.7 Frontal Sinus Surgery (Osteoplastic Flap, Endoscopic Lothrop Procedure)

Indications for surgery [7]:

- Chronic or recurrent frontal sinusitis unresponsive to conservative medical management
- Frontal sinus mucoceles or pyocele
- Frontal sinus fractures with posterior table involvement or cerebrospinal fluid (CSF) leak
- Chronic osteomyelitis of the frontal sinus
- Benign sinonasal tumours involving the frontal sinus

Specific risks involved with the surgery [7]:

- Bleeding
- Infection
- Recurrence of sinus disease
- Injury to adjacent structures (e.g. orbit, skull base, dura)
- Anaesthesia complications
- CSF leak or meningitis (in cases of frontal sinus fracture or skull base involvement)
- Altered facial appearance or contour irregularities

Steps of the surgery:
Osteoplastic flap:

1. Preoperative planning: Obtain imaging studies (e.g. CT scan) to evaluate the extent of sinus disease, anatomy, and any adjacent structure involvement. Discuss the patient's goals and expectations, and develop a surgical plan.
2. Anaesthesia: Administer general anaesthesia.
3. Skin incision: Make a bicoronal or mid-forehead skin incision based on the patient's anatomy and the extent of sinus disease.
4. Flap elevation: Elevate the skin and subcutaneous tissue in the subgaleal or subperiosteal plane, exposing the frontal bone.
5. Osteotomy: Outline an osteotomy around the frontal sinus, preserving the supraorbital rim and the nasal bone. Use a reciprocating saw or chisel to perform the osteotomy, taking care not to damage the posterior table or dura.
6. Sinus debridement: Remove the osteoplastic bone flap, and debride the sinus cavity of any diseased tissue, polyps, or granulation tissue.

7. CSF leak repair (if needed): If a CSF leak is present, repair it using multi-layered reconstruction techniques (e.g. autologous fat graft, fascia lata, synthetic dural substitutes, or vascularized flaps).
8. Sinus obliteration (if indicated): Fill the sinus cavity with an appropriate obliteration material, such as autologous fat, bone graft, or alloplastic materials (e.g. hydroxyapatite cement or bioactive glass).
9. Bone flap replacement and fixation: Replace the osteoplastic bone flap, and secure it in place using miniplates, screws, or sutures.
10. Closure: Close the skin incision in layers, ensuring adequate haemostasis. Apply a head dressing.

Endoscopic Lothrop Procedure:

1. General anaesthesia is used. Total intravenous anaesthesia (TIVA) is preferred for reducing intraoperative/post-operative bleeding. Prepare the nasal cavity with topical decongestants to reduce mucosal bleeding.
2. Administer local anaesthesia with a vasoconstrictor, e.g. 2% lidocaine with 1:80,000 adrenaline (Lignospan©).
3. The patient should be positioned supine on the operating table with their head elevated at about 15°–30°. This head-up position helps reduce venous pressure and minimize bleeding. The patient's head should be stabilized with a headrest, and the surgeon should ensure proper alignment to provide optimal access to the nasal structures.
4. Identify landmarks: Endoscopically visualize the middle turbinate, agger nasi cells, and frontal recess.
5. Frontal sinusotomy: Remove the frontal sinus floor between the middle turbinate and nasal septum, creating a large frontal sinus ostium.
6. Bilateral frontal sinusotomy: If a bilateral procedure is indicated, remove the intersinus septum and the contralateral frontal sinus floor.
7. Sinus debridement: Debride the frontal sinus of any diseased tissue, polyps, or granulation tissue.
8. Post-operative care: Use nasal saline irrigations and topical nasal steroids to promote healing and maintain patency of the frontal sinus ostium.

Important points to note during the surgery:

- Carefully plan the osteotomy to avoid injury to the posterior table or dura and to preserve the supraorbital rim and nasal bone in the osteoplastic flap procedure.
- Ensure thorough debridement of the sinus cavity to minimize the risk of recurrence or persistent infection in both procedures.
- In the endoscopic Lothrop procedure, maintain the patency of the frontal sinus ostium to prevent post-operative stenosis or obstruction.
- Monitor the patient's intraoperative and post-operative condition to detect any complications early and intervene as necessary.

Questions a consultant might ask a trainee about the operation:

1. **How do you decide between an osteoplastic flap procedure and an endoscopic Lothrop procedure for frontal sinus surgery?**
   The choice depends on the extent and location of the sinus disease, the patient's anatomy, and the surgeon's experience and preference. The osteoplastic flap provides better access for sinus obliteration, whereas the endoscopic Lothrop procedure is less invasive and focuses on creating a large frontal sinus ostium for drainage [7].
2. **What are the key anatomic landmarks to identify during an endoscopic Lothrop procedure?**
   Key landmarks include the middle turbinate, agger nasi cells, frontal recess, and frontal sinus floor.
3. **How do you manage a persistent CSF leak after an osteoplastic flap procedure?**
   Persistent CSF leaks can be managed with conservative measures, such as bed rest, elevation of the head, and lumbar drainage. If conservative measures fail, revision surgery with multi-layered reconstruction techniques may be required to repair the leak.
4. **What are the advantages and disadvantages of the osteoplastic flap procedure compared to the endoscopic Lothrop procedure?**
   The osteoplastic flap provides better access for sinus obliteration and may be more effective for managing complex frontal sinus pathology. However, it is more invasive, with a longer recovery time and a higher risk of facial scarring or contour irregularities. The endoscopic Lothrop procedure is less invasive, with minimal scarring and a faster recovery, but may not be suitable for all cases and requires maintaining patency of the frontal sinus ostium post-operatively.

3.8   Septal Perforation Surgery

Indications for surgery [8]:

- Symptomatic septal perforation with crusting, bleeding, nasal obstruction, or whistling despite conservative management
- Saddle nose deformity or cosmetic concerns due to septal perforation

Preoperative Planning:

- Patient assessment: Conduct a comprehensive nasal examination, including anterior rhinoscopy and nasal endoscopy, to evaluate the size, location, and cause of the perforation. Additional investigations, such as a vasculitis screen, can help determine the aetiology of idiopathic septal perforation and exclude contraindications to surgical treatment, such as active vasculitis or cocaine abuse.
- Imaging: Consider a CT scan if there are concerns about sinus involvement or other structural anomalies.

- Conservative management: Attempt conservative management with saline irrigations, emollients, topical antibiotic creams, or use of a septal button, if appropriate.
- Discussion of surgical options: Discuss the risks and benefits of surgical repair versus continued conservative management with the patient.

Risks involved with the surgery [8]:

- Infection
- Septal haematoma
- Adhesions
- Failure of graft and recurrence of septal perforation
- Change in shape of the nose/saddle nose deformity

Steps of surgery:

1. This procedure can be performed via an endonasal, endoscopic, or open septorhinoplasty approach.
2. Administer general anaesthesia: Total intravenous anaesthesia (TIVA) is preferred to reduce intraoperative and post-operative bleeding.
3. Prepare the nasal cavity: Use topical decongestants to reduce mucosal bleeding. Administer local anaesthesia with a vasoconstrictor, such as 2% lidocaine with 1:80,000 adrenaline.
4. Perform incision: Make a hemitransfixion or Killian incision to access the septal cartilage and bone.
5. Elevate flaps: Elevate mucoperichondrial flaps on both sides of the septum to expose the perforation edges.
6. Unilateral flap: In certain cases, a unilateral mucoperichondrial flap may be sufficient if the perforation is small and accessible from one side.
7. Freshen edges: Use a scalpel or scissors to create a raw surface at the perforation edges to facilitate healing.
8. Types of closure:
   - Bipedicle advancement flap:
     – Procedure: Elevate mucoperichondrial and mucoperiosteal flaps from both sides of the septum. These flaps are advanced towards the perforation. The edges of the perforation are freshened to create a raw surface, which promotes healing. The flaps are then meticulously positioned to cover the perforation, ensuring that there is no tension.
     – Indication: Suitable for small- to medium-sized perforations where bilateral mucosal advancement is feasible.
   - Rotational flap:
     – Procedure: Create a rotational mucosal flap from the nasal septum. An incision is made around the perforation, and the flap is rotated into position. An acellular dermal interposition graft, such as Biodesign™, is placed between the flap and the septum to provide structural support and enhance healing. The graft is secured with fine absorbable sutures.

- Indication: Used for larger perforations where a simple advancement flap would not provide sufficient coverage.
- Anterior ethmoidal artery septal flap:
  - Procedure: Begin by identifying the anterior ethmoidal artery. A mucoperichondrial and mucoperiosteal flap is created, based on the artery, to ensure a robust blood supply. This flap is then elevated and advanced to cover the perforation. The edges of the perforation are freshened to facilitate healing, and the flap is secured in place with fine absorbable sutures.
  - Indication: Ideal for large perforations or those located anteriorly, where enhanced vascular supply is crucial for successful healing.
- Facial artery myomucosal flap (FAMM):
  - Procedure: The facial artery is identified, and a myomucosal flap is harvested from the buccal mucosa. This flap is then transposed into the nasal cavity to cover the septal perforation. The robust blood supply from the facial artery helps ensure the viability of the flap and promotes healing.
  - Indication: Suitable for large defects where robust blood supply and coverage are necessary.
- Interposition graft:
  - Procedure: After creating the appropriate mucosal flaps, an interposition graft such as an acellular dermal matrix (e.g. Biodesign™) or auricular cartilage graft is placed between the flaps. This graft provides structural support and facilitates healing by maintaining separation between the flaps. The graft is secured with fine absorbable sutures.
  - Indication: Used to reinforce the repair, particularly in larger perforations or those requiring additional structural support.
- Suture flaps:
  - Procedure: Carefully suture the flaps with fine absorbable sutures, ensuring that the flaps are well apposed with no gaping or tension at the suture lines. This meticulous closure is essential to prevent dehiscence and ensure successful healing.
  - Indication: Applicable to all types of flap repairs to ensure proper closure and healing.
- Septal button:
  - Procedure: If primary closure of the perforation is not feasible, a septal button can be inserted to temporarily alleviate symptoms. This button acts as a physical barrier, reducing symptoms such as whistling and crusting, while further surgical options are considered.
  - Indication: Used as a temporary measure for symptomatic relief when definitive surgical repair is not immediately possible.

Post-operative care:

- Nasal packing or splints: Place soft nasal packing or splints to support the septum, reduce bleeding, and prevent adhesions.

- Follow-up: Schedule post-operative follow-up to monitor the healing process and address any complications such as infection, haematoma, or persistent perforation.
- Patient instructions: Advise the patient on saline irrigations and nasal ointments to keep the nasal mucosa moist and promote healing.

Important Points to Note During Surgery:

- Meticulous dissection: Close to the septum is crucial to avoid damage to adjacent structures and ensure successful repair.
- Proper visualization: Ensure optimal positioning and visualization of the surgical field.
- Intraoperative documentation: Endoscopic photos pre- and post-procedure help in documenting the process and verifying the results.
- Post-operative monitoring: Careful observation for signs of complications, such as infection or haematoma, is essential for early detection and management.

Questions a consultant might ask a trainee during the operation:

1. **What are the potential causes of septal perforations, and how can these influence the surgical approach?**
    Septal perforations can result from trauma (e.g. nasal fracture, nose picking), previous nasal surgeries (e.g. septoplasty), chronic inflammatory diseases (e.g. granulomatosis with polyangiitis), infections, long-term use of nasal decongestants, and intranasal drug use (e.g. cocaine). The underlying cause can influence the surgical approach; for instance, in cases caused by chronic inflammation, ensuring complete removal of inflamed tissue and using well-vascularized flaps are crucial to prevent recurrence. In cases of perforations due to trauma, more robust structural support might be needed.
2. **How does the location and size of the septal perforation affect the choice of flap for repair?**
    The location and size of the perforation are critical in determining the appropriate flap technique. Small perforations (less than 1 cm) can often be repaired using simple advancement flaps. Medium-sized perforations (1–2 cm) might require rotational flaps or bipedicled advancement flaps for adequate coverage. Large perforations (greater than 2 cm), especially those located anteriorly, may necessitate the use of vascularized flaps like the anterior ethmoidal artery flap or the facial artery myomucosal flap (FAMM) due to their robust blood supply, which enhances healing and reduces the risk of recurrence.
3. **Describe the anatomical considerations and steps involved in creating an anterior ethmoidal artery flap for septal perforation repair**
    To create an anterior ethmoidal artery flap for septal perforation repair, start at the posterior aspect of the perforation, ensuring that the flap includes both mucoperichondrium and mucoperiosteum. Make a vertical incision on the septum, 0.5–1.0 cm behind the septal projection of the axilla of the middle turbi-

nate, marking the posterior edge of the flap. Continue the incision along the nasal floor, following the posterior border of the hard palate until it reaches the lateral wall of the posterior part of the inferior meatus. Then, extend the incision parallel to the septum along the lateral border of the inferior meatus until it reaches the anterior section. At this point, make the incision perpendicular to the septum, connecting it to the inferior border of the perforation. Finally, extend the incision into the inferior meatus to create a larger mucosal flap, allowing for tension-free advancement of the flap. These steps ensure that the flap is appropriately sized and positioned for effective septal perforation repair.

4. **What are the advantages and potential complications of using acellular dermal matrix as an interposition graft in septal perforation repair?**

   Advantages of using acellular dermal matrix (ADM) include its biocompatibility, ability to integrate with host tissue, and provision of structural support to the repaired area. ADM also reduces the risk of immunogenic rejection and provides a scaffold for cellular infiltration and vascularization. Potential complications include infection, graft extrusion or rejection, and insufficient integration, which can lead to recurrence of the perforation. Proper handling and positioning of the ADM are crucial to mitigate these risks.

5. **How would you manage a patient presenting with a whistling noise post-operatively, and what could this indicate about the success of the septal perforation repair?**

   A whistling noise post-operatively often indicates a residual or recurrent septal perforation. Initial management includes a thorough nasal examination to confirm the presence and size of the perforation. Conservative measures such as humidification, saline irrigations, and application of emollients can be used to reduce symptoms. If the perforation is symptomatic and persistent, surgical revision may be necessary. The cause of the initial repair failure, such as inadequate flap coverage or poor vascularization, should be identified and addressed in the subsequent procedure.

References

1. Luong A, Marple BF. Sinus surgery: indications and techniques. Clin Rev Allergy Immunol. 2006;30:217–22.
2. Shah J, Roxbury CR, Sindwani R. Techniques in septoplasty: traditional versus endoscopic approaches. Otolaryngol Clin N Am. 2018;51(5):909–17.
3. Batra PS, Seiden AM, Smith TL. Surgical management of adult inferior turbinate hypertrophy: a systematic review of the evidence. Laryngoscope. 2009;119(9):1819–27.
4. Woog JJ, Kennedy RH, Custer PL, Kaltreider SA, Meyer DR, Camara JG. Endonasal dacryocystorhinostomy. Ophthalmology. 2001;108(12):2369–77.
5. Lee SC, Senior BA. Endoscopic skull base surgery. Clin Exp Otorhinolaryngol. 2008;1(2):53–62.
6. Rohrich RJ, Ahmad J. Rhinoplasty. Plast Reconstr Surg. 2011;128(2):49e–73e.
7. Wormald PJ. Salvage frontal sinus surgery: the endoscopic modified Lothrop procedure. Laryngoscope. 2003;113(2):276–83.
8. Watson D, Barkdull G. Surgical management of the septal perforation. Otolaryngol Clin N Am. 2009;42(3):483–93.

Laryngology

Natalie Watson, Zohaib Siddiqui, Basim Wahba, and Keli Dusu

4.1 Microlaryngoscopy (ML)

Indications for surgery [1]:

- Diagnostic evaluation of laryngeal lesions or abnormalities
- Biopsy of laryngeal lesions
- Removal of benign or malignant vocal fold lesions
- Treatment of vocal fold immobility
- Injection of material (e.g. botulinum toxin/steroid/filler) into larynx
- Management of laryngeal stenosis or scarring

Risks involved with the surgery [1]:

- Bleeding
- Infection
- Pain
- Recurrent or residual symptoms
- Injury to the vocal folds, leading to voice changes or hoarseness
- Airway compromise, including laryngospasm or oedema
- Laser airway fire (if laser is used)

N. Watson (✉)
Guy's & St Thomas NHS Foundation Trust, St Thomas' Hospital, London, UK

Z. Siddiqui
Medway NHS Foundation Trust, Gillingham, Kent, UK

B. Wahba
Queen Victoria Hospital, East Grinstead, UK

K. Dusu
Frimley Park Hospital, Camberley, UK

- Migration of injected material (if material is injected)

Steps of the surgery:

1. Administer general anaesthesia, and perform endotracheal intubation with a micro-laryngology tube (MLT). The tube can be placed 26 cm from incisor for females and 28 cm for males; alternatively, ensure that the balloon is sited far enough below the cords in order not to pull up the larynx. Alternatively, this can also be performed tubeless on selected patients using high-flow oxygen (Optiflow) or with jet ventilation.
2. Position the patient supine with the neck in the Boyce-Jackson position with extension at the atlanto-occipital joint and flexion of the neck on the chest. It is also known as 'sniffing the morning air'.
3. Protect the teeth with a mouth guard.
4. Insert a laryngoscope (e.g. Lindholm) to expose the larynx, and once an adequate view is achieved, stabilise the larynx using a laryngeal suspension system as seen in Fig. 4.1.
5. Glottic pressure may be required if an optimum view has not been achieved.
6. Utilise an operating microscope or 0°-, 30°-, or 70° endoscope (Hopkins rod) for enhanced visualisation of the laryngeal structures. Photodocumentation of the findings is then recommended.
7. Perform the planned procedure (e.g. biopsy, lesion removal, vocal fold augmentation) using microsurgical instruments or laser technology.
8. Ensure adequate haemostasis during and after the procedure using adrenaline-soaked gauze.
9. Suction excess or pooled saliva/blood from bronchi/trachea/larynx/pharynx/oral cavity.
10. Remove the laryngoscope or laryngeal suspension system, and extubate the patient, if applicable.
11. Monitor the patient in the recovery room for any complications.

Important points to note during the surgery:

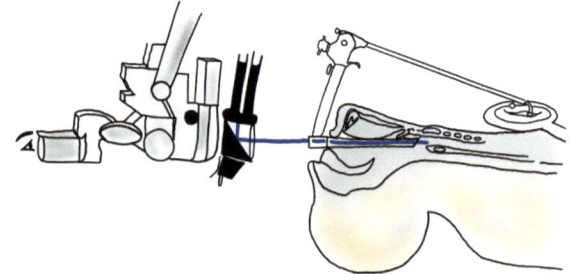

Fig. 4.1 Laryngoscope with suspension system and microscope. (Illustrated by Vikum Liyanaarachchi)

- Gentle handling of laryngeal structures is crucial to prevent injury and preserve vocal function.
- Adequate exposure and visualisation of the laryngeal structures are essential for a successful microlaryngoscopy.
- Try to avoid operating on the vibrating edge of the vocal folds to reduce voice change and chance of strictures/webbing.
- Important not to strip the vocal cord mucosa or take a biopsy through the vocal cord ligament.

Questions a consultant might ask a trainee about the operation:

1. **What are the indications for performing microlaryngoscopy?**
   Indications for performing microlaryngoscopy include the diagnostic evaluation of laryngeal lesions or abnormalities, biopsy of laryngeal lesions, removal of benign or malignant vocal fold lesions, treatment of vocal fold immobility, and management of laryngeal stenosis or scarring [1]. Microlaryngoscopy provides high-resolution visualisation of the laryngeal structures, allowing for precise and minimally invasive surgical interventions.
2. **How do you differentiate between benign and malignant vocal fold lesions?**
   Differentiating between benign and malignant vocal fold lesions often involves a combination of clinical history, endoscopic examination preferably with high-definition images, stroboscopy and narrowband imaging, and histopathological evaluation [1]. Clinically, malignant lesions may present with progressive hoarseness, dysphagia, odynophagia, or referred otalgia. Endoscopically, malignant lesions may appear as irregular, ulcerated, or infiltrating masses, while benign lesions typically present as well-circumscribed, smooth, or polypoid masses. However, the definitive diagnosis is usually made after obtaining a tissue biopsy and performing a histopathological examination, which can reveal features, such as cellular atypia, invasion, and high mitotic activity in malignant lesions.
3. **What are the potential complications of microlaryngoscopy, and how can they be minimised?**
   Potential complications of microlaryngoscopy include haemorrhage, infection, injury to the vocal folds leading to voice changes or hoarseness, recurrent or residual symptoms, and airway compromise, such as laryngospasm or oedema. To minimise complications, surgeons should handle laryngeal structures gently, ensure adequate exposure and visualisation of the laryngeal structures, and achieve meticulous haemostasis. Careful patient selection and thorough preoperative planning are essential to achieving good outcomes.
4. **Can you describe the different types of vocal fold lesions that can be managed with microlaryngoscopy?**
   Several types of vocal fold lesions can be managed with microlaryngoscopy, including [2]:
   - Examples of lesions (Fig. 4.2):
     - Benign lesions: vocal fold polyps, nodules, cysts, granulomas, or papilloma

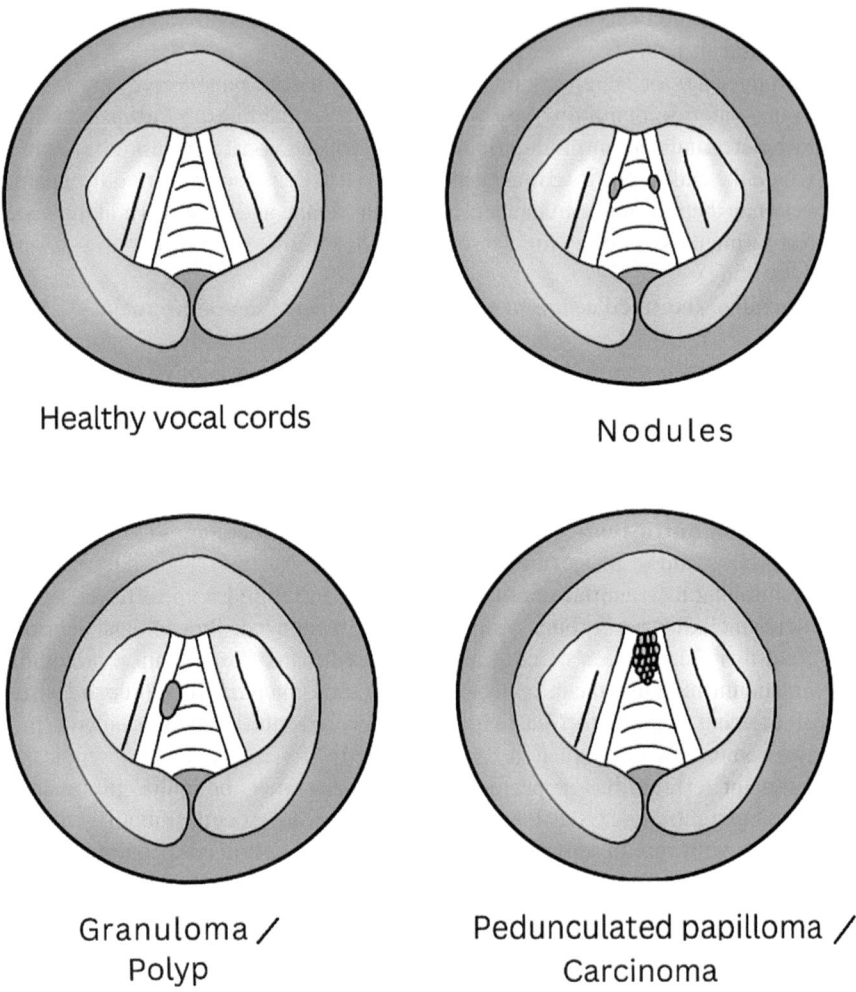

Fig. 4.2 View of larynx with examples of lesions seen. (Illustrated by Vikum Liyanaarachchi)

- Malignant lesions: squamous cell carcinoma (90%), adenocarcinoma, sarcoma, adenoid cystic carcinoma, or other rare malignancies
5. **What are the roles of cold instruments, CO2 laser, and other lasers including potassium-titanyl-phosphate (KTP), green and blue lasers, and laryngeal microdebrider in microlaryngoscopy?**
   All these tools have specific roles in microlaryngoscopy:
   - Cold instruments: These tools provide precise dissection and removal of vocal fold lesions, especially when preservation of the delicate vocal fold tissue is crucial. However, they may be associated with a higher risk of bleeding compared to laser techniques.

- CO_2 laser: The CO_2 laser provides precise cutting and coagulation capabilities with minimal thermal damage to the surrounding tissue. It is particularly useful for the management of early-stage laryngeal cancer, benign lesions such as papillomas, or airway stenosis.
- KTP, green and blue laser: The KTP laser has excellent haemostatic properties and can be used for the treatment of vascular lesions, such as recurrent respiratory papillomatosis or capillary ectasias. It can be applied in a contact or non-contact mode and may also be used in office-based procedures under local anaesthesia.
- A microdebrider can be used to debulk laryngeal papilloma and other bulky lesions with less thermal damage and less risk of viral particle transmission and avoid the potential airway fire risks associated with laser treatment.

6. **What are the prevalent types of laryngoscopes used in practice?**
   - Lindholm laryngoscope: Offers a panoramic view, ideal for inserting into the vallecula to visualise the entire larynx.
   - Rhys-Evans laryngoscope: Suitable for folding the epiglottis or when facing difficult exposure cases where the Lindholm provides inadequate visualisation. Its tip is designed to be placed underneath the epiglottis, though it offers a narrower view.
   - Anterior commissure laryngoscopes (e.g. Hollinger, Negus): Specifically designed for elevating the epiglottic tubercle, facilitating exposure of the anterior commissure.
   - Dedo-Pilling laryngoscope: Effective in challenging exposure scenarios, such as with a short neck or limited jaw opening, and for anterior commissure exposure.
   - Feyh-Kastenbauer (FK) retractor: Primarily used in transoral robotic surgery, with limited application for certain laryngeal lesions.

7. **What are the classification types for transoral laser microsurgery (TLM) in treating glottic cancer, as per the European Laryngological Society [3]?**
   - Type I: subepithelial cordectomy
   - Type II: subligamental cordectomy
   - Type III: transmuscular cordectomy
   - Type IV: complete cordectomy
   - Type Va: extended cordectomy, encompassing contralateral vocal fold
   - Type Vb: extended cordectomy, encompassing an arytenoid resection
   - Type Vc: supraglottic, extended cordectomy encompassing the ventricular fold
   - Type Vd: extended cordectomy, encompassing the subglottis
   - Type VI: extended cordectomy, encompassing the anterior commissure and the anterior part of both vocal cords

4.2 Arytenoidectomy

Indications for surgery [4]:

- Treatment of bilateral vocal fold immobility, particularly abductor paralysis
- Ankylosis of arytenoid cartilages or cricoarytenoid joints, e.g. rheumatoid arthritis
- As part of the management of posterior glottic stenosis
- Decompression of the airway in cases of severe laryngeal obstruction
- Treatment of recurrent laryngeal nerve paralysis

Risks involved with the surgery [4]:

- Bleeding
- Infection
- Aspiration or swallowing difficulties
- Voice changes or hoarseness
- Airway compromise, such as laryngospasm or oedema

Steps of the surgery:

1. Administer general anaesthesia with endotracheal intubation (MLT) or jet ventilation.
2. Position the patient supine with the neck in the Boyce-Jackson position with extension at the atlanto-occipital joint and flexion of the neck on the chest.
3. Perform microlaryngoscopy or direct laryngoscopy to visualise the laryngeal structures. A Dedo or Dedo-Pilling laryngoscope is preferred.
4. Identify the arytenoid cartilage and surrounding structures, including the vocal folds, the aryepiglottic folds, and the posterior commissure.
5. Using cold instruments, a CO_2 laser, a microdebrider, or coblation, carefully dissect and remove the arytenoid cartilage fully or partially, taking care to preserve as much of the surrounding structures as possible. Figure 4.3 highlights the different types of procedures.
6. Achieve meticulous haemostasis using adrenaline-soaked patties or electrocautery. A laryngeal suction monopolar diathermy is useful in this situation.
7. Inspect the surgical site for any residual cartilage or tissue that may obstruct the airway.
8. Close the larynx using absorbable sutures if needed, and remove the laryngoscope.
9. Extubate the patient, and monitor for any signs of airway compromise or other complications.

Important points to note during the surgery:

- Adequate exposure and visualisation of the laryngeal structures are crucial for a successful outcome.
- The procedure should be performed with extreme care and precision to minimise injury to the surrounding structures.

4 Laryngology

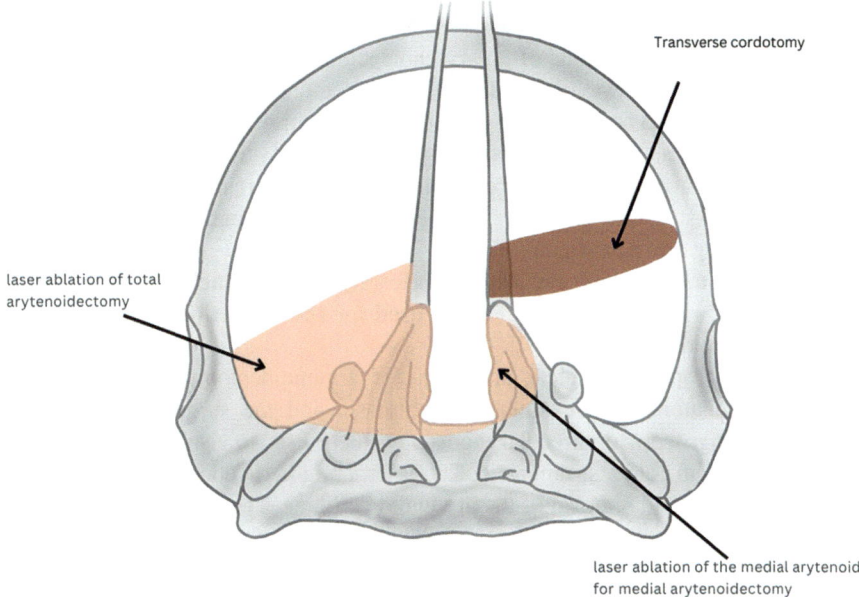

Fig. 4.3 Arytenoidectomy procedures. (Illustrated by Vikum Liyanaarachchi)

- Proper patient selection and thorough preoperative planning, including a comprehensive assessment of the patient's airway, preoperative swallowing, voice status, and overall condition, are essential for achieving successful outcomes.

Questions a consultant might ask a trainee about the operation:

1. **What are the indications for performing an arytenoidectomy?**
   Arytenoidectomy is indicated for the treatment of bilateral vocal fold immobility, particularly abductor paralysis, management of posterior glottic stenosis, decompression of the airway in cases of severe laryngeal obstruction, and treatment of recurrent laryngeal nerve paralysis. The procedure involves the removal of the arytenoid cartilage to widen the airway and improve respiratory function.
2. **Can you describe the anatomy of the arytenoid cartilage and its relationship to the surrounding laryngeal structures?**
   The arytenoid cartilages are a pair of pyramid-shaped structures located on the posterior aspect of the cricoid cartilage. They articulate with the cricoid cartilage through the cricoarytenoid joint and play a crucial role in vocal fold movement. Each arytenoid cartilage has a vocal process that attaches to the vocal ligament and a muscular process that connects to the posterior and lateral cricoarytenoid muscles. The surrounding laryngeal structures include the vocal fold, the aryepiglottic fold, and the posterior commissure.

3. **What are the potential complications of arytenoidectomy, and how can they be minimised?**

    Potential complications of an arytenoidectomy include haemorrhage, infection, aspiration or swallowing difficulties, voice changes, and airway compromise, such as laryngospasm or oedema. To minimise complications, surgeons should ensure adequate exposure and visualisation of the laryngeal structures, perform the procedure with extreme care and precision to minimise injury to the surrounding structures, and carefully select patients through thorough preoperative planning and assessment.

4. **How do you determine the appropriate surgical approach for arytenoidectomy, and what instruments can be used for the dissection and removal of the arytenoid cartilage?**

    The appropriate surgical approach for arytenoidectomy depends on the patient's anatomy, the extent of the disease, and the surgeon's experience. Microlaryngoscopy or direct laryngoscopy can be used to visualise the laryngeal structures, and cold instruments, a CO_2 laser, or a microdebrider can be used for the dissection and removal of the arytenoid cartilage. The choice of instruments depends on the surgeon's preference, the availability of equipment, and the specific clinical situation.

5. **What are the different techniques of arytenoidectomy?**

    Arytenoidectomy, a surgical procedure aimed at removing part or all of an arytenoid cartilage, can be performed using several techniques, each with specific indications, benefits, and limitations. These techniques can be broadly categorised into intralaryngeal (often performed using microlaryngoscopy and lasers) and extralaryngeal approaches.

    Intralaryngeal (Microlaryngoscopic) Techniques
    - Laser transverse posterior cordotomy (Kashima procedure): This involves making an incision anterior to the vocal process using a laser. The technique aims to enlarge the glottic space without exposing the cartilage, preserving vocal quality while improving breathing.
    - Laser medial arytenoidectomy: This procedure entails the precise removal of the medial aspect of the arytenoid cartilage using laser technology, which can help in cases where vocal fold mobility is significantly impaired, but aims to minimise the impact on the swallow mechanism.
    - Laser posterior cordotomy with partial arytenoidectomy: It combines the removal of a portion of the arytenoid cartilage with a posterior cordotomy. This approach is used to address bilateral vocal fold paralysis by widening the airway while attempting to preserve voice quality in addition to swallow.
    - Endoscopic suture lateralisation: This technique involves the lateral repositioning of the vocal fold through suturing, rather than removing arytenoid cartilage, to improve the airway in cases of paralysis.
    - Extralaryngeal Approaches
    - Type II thyroplasty (lateralisation): Also known as Woodman's procedure, this older method involves external manipulation and lateralisation of the arytenoid cartilage through a surgical approach, often accompanied by suturing

4 Laryngology

of the vocal process laterally. It is aimed at improving the airway in cases where intralaryngeal approaches may not be feasible or preferred.

6. **What are the boundaries of the larynx and its divisions?**

    The larynx, stretching from the base of the tongue to the trachea, is anatomically divided into three distinct regions: the supraglottis, glottis, and subglottis, each with its own unique structures and boundaries.

    - **Supraglottis**: Occupying the upper portion just above the glottis, this area includes the epiglottis, aryepiglottic folds, and arytenoids. Its boundaries stretch from the tip of the epiglottis down to the laryngeal ventricle, marking a space or recess within the larynx.
    - **Glottis**: Positioned in the middle, this region encompasses the vocal folds (true vocal cords) and the rima glottidis (space between the vocal folds). The glottis extends from where the middle one-third and lower one-third of the vocal fold meet, down to 1 cm below the free edge of the vocal fold. This area is crucial for voice production, with its boundaries defined both anatomically by the true vocal cords and functionally by the space they encompass.
    - **Subglottis**: Located below the glottis, extending down to the trachea, the subglottis begins just beneath the vocal folds and continues to the lower border of the cricoid cartilage, marking the end of the larynx and the start of the trachea.

4.3 Vocal Fold Augmentation

Indications for surgery [5]:

- Unilateral vocal fold paralysis or paresis
- Vocal fold atrophy
- Glottic insufficiency (incomplete closure of the vocal folds)
- Scarred or stiff vocal folds
- Sulcus vocalis (groove in the vocal fold)

Risks involved with the surgery [5]:

- Over- or under-injection of the material, leading to inadequate or excessive augmentation
- Infection
- Haematoma
- Allergic reaction to the injected material
- Migration of the injected material
- Granuloma formation
- Airway obstruction (rare)

Steps of the surgery:

1. Administer local anaesthesia with or without sedation, or general anaesthesia, depending on the patient's clinical condition and surgeon's preference.
2. Visualise the larynx using a laryngoscope or a flexible nasopharyngoscopy.
3. If using a transoral approach, insert an endoscope to visualise the vocal folds.
4. Identify the target site for injection, typically at the medial aspect of the vocal process or the mid-membranous portion of the vocal fold.
5. Prepare the chosen augmentation material (e.g. autologous fat, hyaluronic acid, calcium hydroxyapatite, or other synthetic materials).
6. Aspirate the material into a syringe with a small-gauge needle.
7. Inject the material into the vocal fold, either through a transoral or a transcutaneous approach (cricothyroid or thyrohyoid), depending on the surgeon's preference and experience. See Figs. 4.4 and 4.5 for anatomy and position of injection.

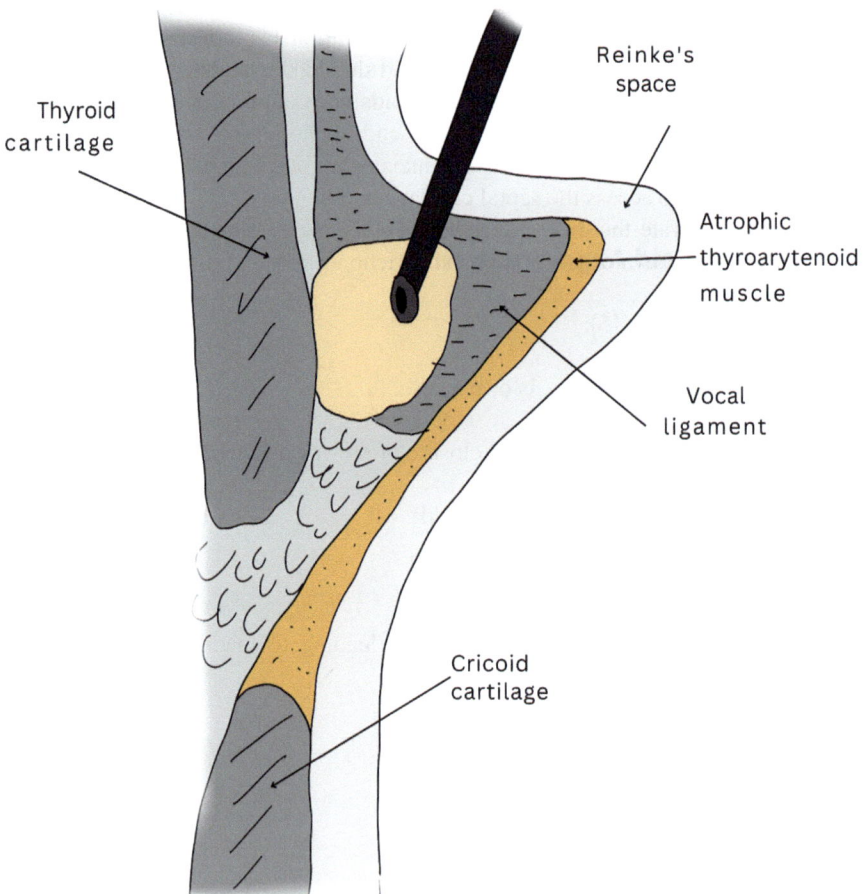

Fig. 4.4 Vocal cord medialisation injection anatomy. (Illustrated by Vikum Liyanaarachchi)

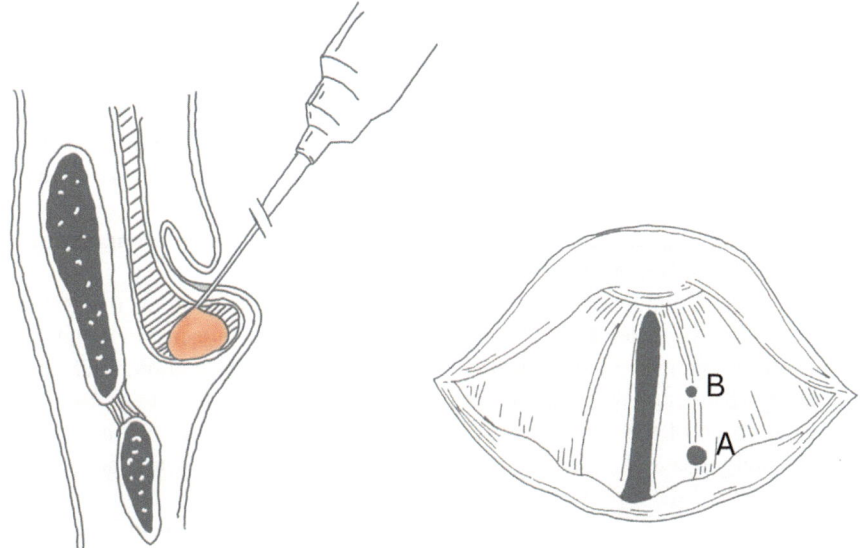

Fig. 4.5 Vocal cord medialisation injection position. (Illustrated by Vikum Liyanaarachchi)

8. Periodically assess the vocal fold closure and phonation during the procedure to determine the adequacy of augmentation, if under local anaesthetic.
9. Once the desired vocal fold position and closure are achieved, remove the instruments and complete the procedure.

Important points to note during the surgery:

- Proper visualisation of the vocal folds is essential for accurate injection and optimal outcomes.
- The choice of augmentation material depends on factors, such as the surgeon's preference, patient's needs, and expected duration of the effect.
- Adequate augmentation should be achieved while avoiding over-injection, which may lead to breathy voice, difficulty swallowing, or airway obstruction.

Questions a consultant might ask a trainee about the operation:

1. **What are the indications for vocal fold augmentation?**
   The indications for vocal fold augmentation include unilateral vocal fold paralysis or paresis, vocal fold atrophy, glottic insufficiency (incomplete closure of the vocal folds), scarred or stiff vocal folds, and sulcus vocalis (a groove in the vocal fold). Vocal fold augmentation aims to improve voice quality, swallowing function, and cough efficiency by optimising vocal fold closure [5].
2. **Can you describe the anatomy of the vocal folds and the surrounding laryngeal structures?**

The vocal folds, also known as vocal cords, are located within the larynx and consist of a multi-layered structure including the epithelium, superficial lamina propria, intermediate lamina propria, deep lamina propria, and vocalis muscle. The vocal folds are responsible for voice production through vibration during phonation. The surrounding laryngeal structures include the thyroid cartilage, cricoid cartilage, arytenoid cartilages, and epiglottis, which all play a role in the complex function of the larynx.

3. **What are the potential complications of vocal fold augmentation, and how can they be minimised?**

   Potential complications of vocal fold augmentation include over- or under-injection of the material, infection, allergic reaction to the injected material, haematoma, migration of the injected material, granuloma formation, and, rarely, airway obstruction. To minimise complications, surgeons should ensure proper visualisation of the vocal folds, choose an appropriate augmentation material, accurately inject the material to achieve optimal vocal fold closure, and closely monitor the patient post-operatively.

4. **What other surgical options are available for treating vocal fold immobility or glottic insufficiency?**

   Other surgical options for treating vocal fold immobility or glottic insufficiency include medialisation thyroplasty (placing an implant to medialise the paralysed vocal fold), arytenoid adduction (suturing the arytenoid cartilage to improve vocal fold closure), laryngeal reinnervation (reconnecting nerves to restore vocal fold function), and, in some cases, laryngeal framework surgery or laser surgery to reshape or reposition the vocal folds. The choice of surgical intervention depends on factors, such as the underlying cause of the vocal fold dysfunction, patient's clinical condition, and surgeon's experience and preference.

5. **What materials are used for vocal cord augmentation in unilateral vocal cord palsy through injection laryngoplasty?**

   Materials for injection laryngoplasty (IL) can be divided into absorbable and non-absorbable categories [5]:
   - Absorbable materials:
     – Short term:
     – Collagen
     – Hyaluronic acid
   - Long term:
     – Calcium hydroxyapatite (CaHA): durable and stable, with a potential risk of granuloma formation
     – Autologous fat: requires more invasive harvesting with variable resorption rates
     – Autologous fascia
     – Poly-dimethyl-siloxane (bioplastique or VOX)
   - Non-absorbable materials:
     – Teflon

- Silicone: These materials have a higher likelihood of causing reactions or granulomas.
6. **What are the approaches for injection laryngoplasty and preferred injection sites?**
   - Transcutaneous (cricothyroid, thyrohyoid, or trans-cartilaginous approaches)
   - Transoral
   - Microlaryngoscopic

   Injection sites: The augmentation material is typically injected lateral to the vocal cord in the paraglottic space, starting from the vocal process. This method aims to close mid and posterior glottic gaps. Additional material may also be injected lateral to the mid-vocal cord for improved closure.
7. **What are the layers of the vocal cord?**
   The vocal cords are structured into several distinct layers, each contributing to vocal cord vibration and voice production:
   Superficial vibratory gelatinous layer:
   - Squamous epithelium
   - Subepithelial: Reinke's space
   - Superficial lamina propria

   Ligamentous layer:
   - Intermediate lamina propria
   - Deep lamina propria

   Muscular layer:
   - Thyroarytenoid muscle

   Vocalis muscle: This is medial portion of the thyroarytenoid muscle.

4.4 Thyroplasty (Types I, II, III, IV)

Thyroplasty described by Isshiki:

- Type I: medialisation: unilateral vocal fold paralysis or paresis
- Type II: lateralisation: vocal fold overclosure, abductor spasmodic dysphonia
- Type III: shortening, relaxation (lower pitch): vocal fold underclosure, adductor spasmodic dysphonia
- Type IV: lengthening, tension (raise pitch): vocal fold scar, sulcus, or atrophy

Risks involved with the surgery [6]:

- Haemorrhage
- Infection
- Unintended changes in voice quality
- If used, implant extrusion, migration, or rejection
- Need for revision surgery

Steps of the surgery (e.g. type I thyroplasty):

1. Administer local anaesthesia with or without sedation or general anaesthesia, depending on the patient's clinical condition and surgeon's preference.
2. If under general anaesthetic, position the patient supine with a shoulder roll to extend the neck.
3. Otherwise, if under local anaesthetic, position the patient at 45° so that the patient is comfortable.
4. Mark the incision site on a relaxed skin tension line transversely, 5 cm midline to lateral between the upper border of the thyroid cartilage and cricoid cartilage upper border.
5. Inject local anaesthetic of choice, preferably mixed with adrenaline to the neck.
6. Carefully spray local anaesthetic and decongestant to the nasal cavity in order to view the larynx during the operation with a flexible nasolaryngoendoscope.
7. Make the horizontal skin incision, and dissect through the subcutaneous tissue.
8. Retract the strap muscles laterally to expose the thyroid cartilage fully.
9. This step may differ depending on your implant; however, one method is measuring the height of thyroid cartilage measure and surface mark the level of the vocal cords on the affected thyroid lamina at half the total height from the inferior border of thyroid cartilage. A 12 × 6 mm rectangular window is marked 7 mm lateral to midline and midway between upper and lower thyroid cartilage borders.
10. Create a window in the thyroid cartilage using a 1 mm fissure burr drill or a small osteotome, preserving the inner perichondrium.
11. Insert the implant (e.g. silicone, GORE-TEX, VOIS, or other synthetic materials) through the cartilage window to medialise the paralysed vocal fold. See Fig. 4.6 for examples of impants.
12. Adjust the implant position to optimise vocal fold closure and phonation.
13. Secure the implant in place with sutures, if necessary, e.g. Vicryl 3/0 subcutaneous and skin 5/0 Prolene interrupted sutures.
14. You may decide to close with or without a drain, ensuring proper haemostasis prior to closure.

Important points to note during the surgery:

- Proper patient positioning and exposure of the thyroid cartilage are crucial for successful thyroplasty.
- Careful dissection and measurement for the window are essential to avoid complications and correct placement.
- Continuous assessment of vocal fold closure and phonation is necessary to achieve optimal outcomes.

Questions a consultant might ask a trainee about the operation:

1. **What are the indications for each type of thyroplasty (types I, II, III, IV)?**
   The indications for each type of thyroplasty are as follows:

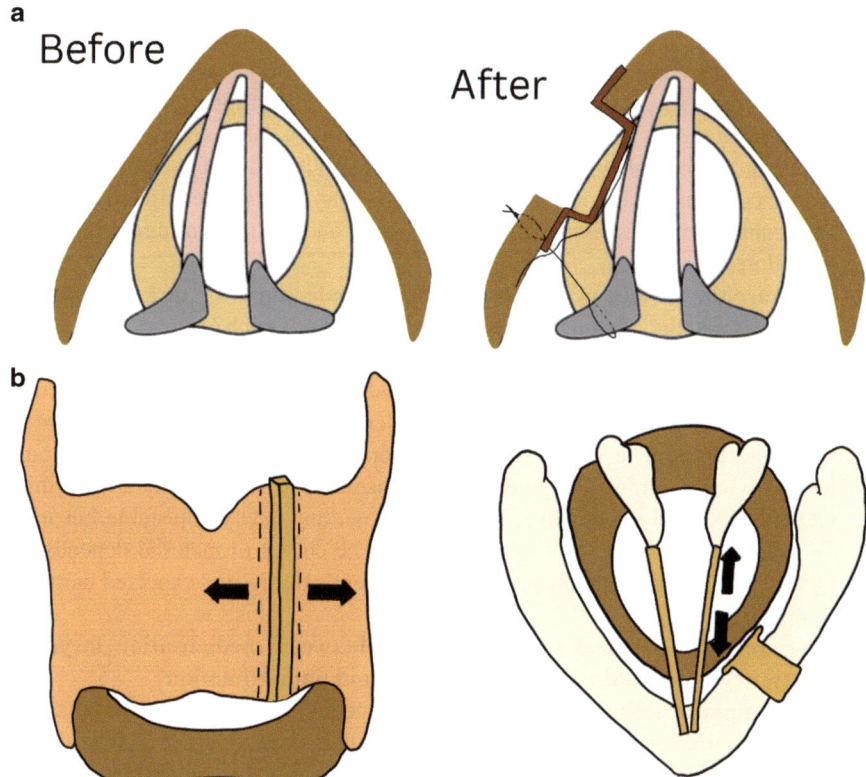

Fig. 4.6 Thyroplasty implant examples. (**a**) Showing left-sided vocal cord palsy in lateral position with implant placed on the left. (**b**) Type II thyroplasty example. (Illustrated by Vikum Liyanaarachchi)

- Type I: Unilateral vocal fold paralysis or paresis; it aims to medialise the paralysed vocal fold, improving voice quality and glottal closure.
- Type II: Vocal fold overclosure, abductor spasmodic dysphonia; it involves lateralising one or both vocal folds to reduce hyperadduction and improve voice quality.
- Type III: Vocal fold underclosure, adductor spasmodic dysphonia; it medialises one or both vocal folds to improve glottal closure and voice quality.
- Type IV: Vocal fold scar, sulcus, or atrophy; it aims to augment the vocal fold by injecting fat, collagen, or other materials to improve voice quality.

2. **Can you describe the anatomy of the larynx and the structures involved in thyroplasty?**

   The larynx is a complex structure located in the neck, responsible for voice production, swallowing, and airway protection. Key laryngeal structures involved in thyroplasty include the thyroid cartilage, cricoid cartilage, arytenoid cartilages, and vocal folds.

3. **What are the potential complications of thyroplasty, and how can they be minimised?**

   Potential complications of thyroplasty include haemorrhage, infection, unintended changes in voice quality, implant extrusion, migration, or rejection, and the need for revision surgery. To minimise complications, surgeons should ensure proper patient positioning, carefully dissect and identify anatomical landmarks, perform meticulous haemostasis, choose an appropriate implant material, and continuously assess vocal fold closure and phonation throughout the procedure.

4. **What are the various materials used for medialisation in type I thyroplasty, and what are the advantages and disadvantages of each?**

   Various materials can be used for medialisation in type I thyroplasty, including silicone, VOIS implant, GORE-TEX, and other synthetic materials. Silicone is biocompatible, easy to shape, and well tolerated but may become encapsulated by fibrous tissue. The VOIS implant is customisable, and one can adjust the balloon size under ultrasound guidance post-insertion percutaneously at any time. GORE-TEX is biocompatible, non-absorbable, and easily adjustable but may require more complex suturing techniques. The choice of material depends on factors, such as the surgeon's preference, patient's needs, and expected duration of the effect.

5. **How does the surgical technique differ between medialisation laryngoplasty, arytenoid adduction, and cricothyroid approximation?**

   The surgical techniques differ between medialisation laryngoplasty, arytenoid adduction, and cricothyroid approximation:
   - Medialisation laryngoplasty: Medialises the paralysed vocal fold by inserting an implant through a window created in the thyroid cartilage. This procedure focuses on medialising the anterior and middle portions of the vocal fold.
   - Arytenoid adduction: Involves the placement of sutures through the muscular process of the arytenoid cartilage and the thyroid cartilage to medialise the posterior portion of the vocal fold. This procedure may be combined with medialisation laryngoplasty for complete vocal fold medialisation.
   - Cricothyroid approximation: Involves suturing the cricoid cartilage to the thyroid cartilage, increasing the tension on the vocal folds, and improving voice quality in patients with vocal fold atrophy, scarring, or other causes of glottic insufficiency.

References

1. Smith J, Johnson A, Lee R. Iowa head and neck protocols. Microdirect laryngoscopy (suspension microlaryngoscopy or direct laryngoscopy. 2023. https://medicine.uiowa.edu/iowaprotocols/microlaryngoscopy.
2. Lehmann W, Pampurik J, Guyot JP. Laryngeal pathologies observed in microlaryngoscopy. ORL. 1989;51(4):206–15.

3. Remacle M, Eckel HE, Antonelli A, Brasnu D, Chevalier D, Friedrich G, et al. Endoscopic cordectomy. A proposal for a classification by the working committee, European laryngological society. Eur Arch Otorrinolaringol. 2000;257(4):227–31. https://doi.org/10.1007/s004050050228.
4. Wani MK, Yarber R, Rosen C, Hengesteg A, Woodson GE. Endoscopic laser medial arytenoidectomy versus total arytenoidectomy in the management of bilateral vocal fold paralysis. Ann Otol Rhinol Laryngol. 1996;105(11):857–62.
5. Siu J, Tam S, Fung K. A comparison of outcomes in interventions for unilateral vocal fold paralysis: a systematic review. Laryngoscope. 2016;126(7):1616–24.
6. Valley ZA, Karp A, Garber D. Safety and adverse events of medialization thyroplasty: a systematic review. Laryngoscope. 2024;134(5):1994–2004.

Paediatrics

Kiran Varadharajan, Zohaib Siddiqui, Basim Wahba, and Keli Dusu

5.1 Adenoidectomy

Indications for Surgery [1]

- Obstructive sleep apnoea due to enlarged adenoids
- Adenoid hypertrophy causing nasal obstruction or mouth breathing (see Fig. 5.1)
- Chronic otitis media with effusion (usually an adjuvant procedure with ventilation tubes)
- Recurrent acute otitis media (usually an adjuvant procedure with ventilation tubes)
- Recurrent or chronic adenoid infection

Specific Risks Involved with the Surgery [1]

- Bleeding
- Infection
- Anaesthesia complications

K. Varadharajan (✉)
Royal Surrey County Hospital, Guildford, Surrey, UK
e-mail: kiranvaradharajan@nhs.net

Z. Siddiqui
Medway NHS Foundation Trust, Gillingham, Kent, UK

B. Wahba
Queen Victoria Hospital, East Grinstead, West Sussex, UK

K. Dusu
Frimley Park Hospital, Frimley, Camberley, UK

© The Author(s), under exclusive license to Springer Nature Switzerland AG 2024
Z. Siddiqui et al. (eds.), *Essentials of ENT Surgical Procedures*,
https://doi.org/10.1007/978-3-031-71394-1_5

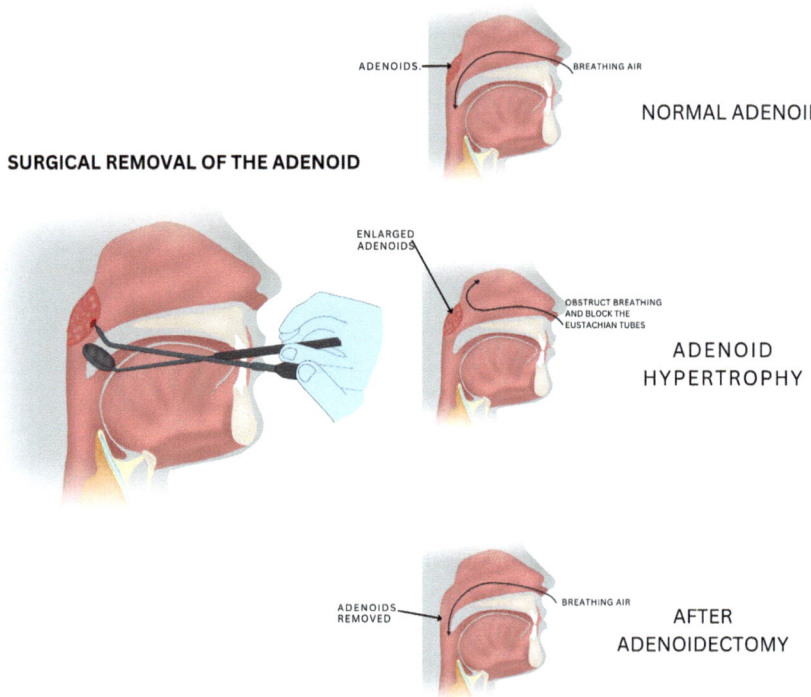

Fig. 5.1 Adenoidectomy before and after. Illustrated by Vikum Liyanaarachchi

- Injury to adjacent structures (e.g. uvula, soft palate, teeth, lips, gum, temporomandibular joint)
- Eustachian tube injury
- Velopharyngeal insufficiency
- Nasopharyngeal stenosis

Steps of the Surgery

1. Anaesthesia: Administer general anaesthesia with an oral endotracheal intubation or laryngeal mask.
2. Positioning: Place a bag/bolster beneath the shoulders of the patient for head extension to expose the nasopharynx.
3. Visualization: Insert a mouth gag to keep the mouth open and soft nasal catheter to elevate the soft palate and visualize the nasopharynx indirectly using a headlight and laryngeal mirror. Check for signs of submucous cleft (bifid uvula, zona pellucida, and hard palate notch).

4. Adenoidectomy: a. Using monopolar suction diathermy or coblation (curettage with a St. Clair Thomson adenoid curette), remove the adenoids by ablating the tissue from the nasopharyngeal wall. c. Ensure complete removal of the adenoid tissue while avoiding injury to surrounding structures (Eustachian tube cushions, septum, turbinates). Pay special attention to remove tissue up-to the choanae which likely contributes most to the nasal blockage. Also avoid injury to Eustachian tube cushions.
5. Haemostasis: Achieve haemostasis by using energy device or packing the nasopharynx with gauze or haemostatic agents, if necessary.
6. Inspection: Inspect the nasopharynx for any remaining adenoid tissue and ensure adequate haemostasis. Ensure clear visualization of the choanae and posterior nasal septum.
7. Recovery: Remove any packing from the nasopharynx, and extubate the patient. Monitor the patient in the recovery room for any complications, such as bleeding or respiratory distress.

Important Points to Note During the Surgery

- Ensure proper patient positioning and exposure of the nasopharynx for adequate visualization.
- Use caution when removing adenoid tissue to avoid injury to the Eustachian tube openings or excessive removal of the underlying nasopharyngeal mucosa.
- Achieve adequate haemostasis to minimize the risk of post-operative bleeding.
- Document if the patient has a bifid uvula as they may have velopharyngeal insufficiency or submucosal cleft palate. If adenoids are removed, the patient may end up with a hypernasal voice.
- In cases of a submucous cleft/previous cleft palate, a superior adenoidectomy is performed (whereby the tissue adjacent to the choanae and away from the palate is targeted to avoid causing problems with velopharyngeal insufficiency).

Questions a Consultant Might Ask a Trainee About the Operation

1. **How do you differentiate between the adenoid tissue and the surrounding structures during the surgery?**
   Adenoid tissue is characterized by its irregular, lobulated appearance and is located in the nasopharynx, posterior to the nasal cavity. To differentiate it from surrounding structures, visualize key landmarks such as the Eustachian tube openings and the torus tubarius. This helps avoid injury to these structures during the procedure.
2. **What are the advantages of using monopolar suction diathermy or coblation techniques in adenoidectomy compared to the traditional curette method?**
   Monopolar suction diathermy and coblation techniques offer superior haemostasis, reducing the risk of post-operative bleeding [1]. These techniques allow

dissection under direct vision, providing a more controlled and precise removal of adenoid tissue. This minimizes the risk of residual tissue and recurrence, enhancing overall surgical outcomes.

3. **What is the role of preoperative imaging in adenoidectomy?**

   Preoperative imaging, such as flexible nasendoscopy, is useful for directly visualizing the adenoids and assessing their size and position. Alternatively, an X-ray of the postnasal space can be used, although it is often not required. Imaging helps in surgical planning and ensures a comprehensive assessment of the adenoid tissue.

4. **How do you manage post-operative bleeding after adenoidectomy?**

   Post-operative bleeding can be managed by applying direct pressure to the nasopharynx, using suction diathermy for cauterization, and repacking the nasopharynx with gauze. Administer intravenous fluids and blood products if necessary to stabilize the patient. Monitoring and timely intervention are crucial to control bleeding effectively.

5. **Define Grisel syndrome and its management.**

   Grisel syndrome is a non-traumatic subluxation of the atlantoaxial joint caused by inflammation of the surrounding ligaments, leading to ligamentous laxity. This condition can trigger muscle spasms and result in torticollis (twisted neck). Management includes immobilization of the neck, anti-inflammatory medications, muscle relaxants, and, in severe cases, surgical intervention to stabilize the joint. Grisel syndrome can be classified into stages based on the degree of subluxation:
   - Stage I: Atlantoaxial rotatory fixation without anterior displacement
   - Stage II: Atlantoaxial rotatory fixation with anterior displacement of 3–5 mm
   - Stage III: Atlantoaxial rotatory fixation with anterior displacement of more than 5 mm
   - Stage IV: Atlantoaxial rotatory fixation with posterior displacement

6. **How do you identify signs of a submucous cleft? Would you proceed with surgery?**

   Signs of a submucous cleft include a bifid uvula, zona pellucida (a thin, translucent line in the midline of the soft palate), and a notch in the hard palate. It is advisable not to proceed with adenoidectomy in these patients due to the high risk of velopharyngeal incompetence. If adenoidectomy is significantly indicated due to severe symptoms, a partial adenoidectomy can be considered after discussing the risks with the patient and their family.

7. **What precautions need to be taken in children with trisomy 21 when performing adenoidectomy?**

   Avoid over-extension of the neck, as children with Down syndrome (trisomy 21) may have atlantoaxial instability in 7–27% of cases. Preoperative screening for cervical spine abnormalities is recommended to minimize the risk of spinal cord injury during surgery.

8. **What is the role of adenoidectomy in otitis media with effusion (OME)?**

   According to NICE guidelines (August 2023), when planning grommets for the management of OME, consider adjuvant adenoidectomy unless assessment indicates an abnormality with the palate [2]. Adenoidectomy can help reduce the incidence of OME by improving Eustachian tube function and decreasing nasopharyngeal obstruction.

9. **What is velopharyngeal insufficiency (VPI), and how does it impact patients?**
Velopharyngeal insufficiency (VPI) is a condition where there is inadequate closure of the velopharyngeal sphincter (the soft palate muscle ring) during speech, resulting in air escaping through the nose. This causes hypernasal speech and can lead to articulation problems, making it difficult for patients to speak clearly. VPI can also affect swallowing, leading to nasal regurgitation of liquids.

5.2 Tonsillectomy

Indications for Surgery [1]

- Recurrent tonsillitis
- Obstructive sleep apnoea due to tonsillar hypertrophy
- Peritonsillar abscess (after the acute phase)
- Suspected malignancy or unexplained unilateral tonsillar enlargement
- Chronic tonsilloliths causing symptoms
- Treatment of a pre-styloid parapharyngeal abscess via an intra-oral approach
- Periodic fever aphthous stomatitis, pharyngitis, and adenitis (PFAPA syndrome)

Specific Risks Involved with the Surgery [1]

- Bleeding
  - 8% overall—5.7% in children, 13% in adults—GIRFT 2019, coblation offers a significantly lower bleeding risk in children.
- Infection
- Anaesthesia complications
- Injury to adjacent structures (e.g. uvula, soft palate, teeth, lips, gum, temporomandibular joint)
- Velopharyngeal insufficiency
- Post-operative pain

Steps of the Surgery (Extra-Capsular)

1. Anaesthesia: Administer general anaesthesia with endotracheal intubation or laryngeal mask.
2. Positioning: Place the patient in the supine position with the head extended using a shoulder bag/bolster.
3. Visualization: Insert a mouth gag to keep the mouth open and visualize the oropharynx using a headlight or operating microscope.
4. Extra-capsular tonsillectomy: (a) Grasp the tonsil with forceps or a snare, and retract medially. (b) Incise the mucosa along the anterior tonsillar pillar using a

scalpel, electrocautery, or coblation device. (c) Dissect the tonsil from the surrounding tissues, including the tonsillar fossa and muscular bed, using a combination of sharp and blunt dissection. (d) Control bleeding using electrocautery, sutures, or haemostatic agents. (e) Repeat the procedure on the contralateral side.
5. Haemostasis: Achieve meticulous haemostasis by applying direct pressure, using electrocautery, or placing sutures, if necessary.
6. Inspection: Inspect the tonsillar fossae to ensure complete removal of tonsillar tissue and adequate haemostasis.
7. Apply topical local anaesthetic with tonsil swabs to the raw tonsil fossae. Then release the mouth gag for up to 3 min. When the gag is engaged again, check for any further bleeding, and remove the tonsil swabs.
8. Suction the postnasal space using a nasal catheter/Yankauer suction to prevent blood clots occluding the airway on extubation.
9. Check for teeth, lip, or gum damage, and check for temporomandibular joint dislocation.
10. Recovery: Extubate the patient and monitor in the recovery room for any complications, such as bleeding or respiratory distress.

Intracapsular Tonsillectomy: All the above steps are the same, except for step 4. The procedure itself is performed from medial to lateral on the tonsil tissue, as seen in Fig. 5.2. The majority of the tonsil tissue is removed, but the capsule is preserved. This is usually done with radiofrequency ablation (e.g. Coblation ®); however, some units use other tools such as the microdebrider. The tonsil tissue is debulked until the capsule is reached, with care not to breach the capsule. Haemostasis is then achieved, and the procedure is repeated on the contralateral

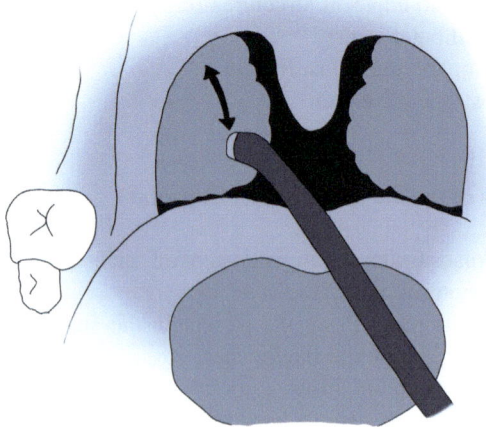

Fig. 5.2 Coblation tonsillectomy. Illustrated by Vikum Liyanaarachchi

side. This procedure is becoming increasingly common for children, especially for those with obstructive sleep apnoea.

Important Points to Note During the Surgery

- Proper visualization and exposure of the tonsils are crucial for a successful procedure.
- Use caution when dissecting the tonsil to minimize injury to surrounding structures, such as the uvula and soft palate.
- Achieve meticulous haemostasis to minimize the risk of post-operative bleeding.

Questions a Consultant Might Ask a Trainee About the Operation

1. **What are the main techniques for tonsillectomy, and what are their advantages and disadvantages?**
    - Tonsillectomy can be performed via extracapsular or intracapsular dissection.
    - The main techniques for extracapsular tonsillectomy include cold steel dissection, electrocautery (bipolar and monopolar), ultrasonic dissection, and coblation. Some also offer laser.
    - The main techniques for intracapsular tonsillectomy/tonsillotomy include coblation and microdebrider.
    - Cold steel dissection is the traditional method with a low rate of thermal injury to surrounding tissues but may have an increased risk of bleeding.
    - Electrocautery provides good haemostasis but may cause more thermal injury and post-operative pain.
    - Ultrasonic dissection also provides good haemostasis with minimal thermal injury (less pain) but requires specialized equipment.
    - Coblation uses radiofrequency energy to produce plasma field using salt water (saline) and has the advantage of minimal thermal injury (less pain) with good haemostasis, but it may be slower and requires specialized equipment. Coblation can be used for both extracapsular and intracapsular dissection. There is a low risk of regrowth of tonsil tissue as you do not remove the capsule.
    - GIRFT study (2019) concluded that intracapsular coblation offers promise for improving outcomes for paediatric tonsillectomy when it is performed in a standardized manner in high volumes with appropriate training and expertise. This is due to the reduced analgesia requirement and lower bleeding rate found in this cohort.
2. **How can you reduce the pain felt from a tonsillectomy?**
    Pain can be managed with a multimodal approach, including the use of long-acting topical anaesthetics (intraoperatively) and systemic analgesics. If there is no contraindication, paracetamol, ibuprofen, and PRN oramorph (side effects of nausea/vomiting/constipation) can be given. Topical antiseptic/anaesthetic sprays, e.g. Difflam©, and non-pharmacologic measures (such as cold therapy and ensuring adequate hydration) can also be used. Codeine and dihydrocodeine are contraindicated in children.

3. How do you differentiate between primary and secondary post-tonsillectomy bleeding, and how do you manage them?

   Primary post-tonsillectomy bleeding occurs within the first 24 h after surgery, while secondary bleeding occurs more than 24 h post-operatively. Primary bleeding is often due to inadequate intraoperative haemostasis and can be managed by re-exploration of the surgical site, direct pressure, electrocautery, or suturing. Secondary bleeding is usually due to infection or sloughing of the eschar and may be managed conservatively or with surgical intervention, depending on the severity and underlying cause.

4. **What precautions should be taken to prevent post-tonsillectomy infection?**

   To prevent post-tonsillectomy infection, ensure strict aseptic technique during the surgery, consider administering perioperative antibiotics, and educate the patient on proper post-operative care, including maintaining good oral hygiene, avoiding spicy or hard foods, and using saline gargles.

5. **What is the significance of the tonsillar capsule, and how is it relevant to the surgical technique?**

   The tonsillar capsule is a thin layer of fibrous tissue that separates the tonsil from the underlying pharyngeal muscles. Preserving the capsule during dissection can minimize injury to surrounding structures, reduce post-operative pain, and lower the risk of bleeding. Different surgical techniques may involve varying degrees of dissection along the capsule, depending on the surgeon's preference and the specific patient's anatomy.

6. **A child needs to go back to theatre for arrest of post-tonsillectomy bleeding. What measures intraoperatively are to be considered, and what could be done to stop the bleeding?**

   - Rapid sequence anaesthesia: Secure the airway with rapid sequence induction to minimize the risk of aspiration. Ensure gastric emptying if necessary.
   - Topical application of tranexamic acid and adrenaline to promote clot formation and reduce bleeding.
   - Haemostasis techniques:
     – Bipolar diathermy: Use bipolar diathermy to cauterize the bleeding vessels.
     – Suture ligation: Directly ligate the bleeding pedicle.
     – Suturing the tonsillar bed: Suture the tonsillar pillars together with a dissolvable haemostatic packing agent to control diffuse bleeding.
     – If bleeding is intractable:
   (a) Activate the major haemorrhage protocol. This involves transfusion of blood products and volume resuscitation.
   (b) Apply a pack sutured over the tonsil fossa to control bleeding.
   (c) Keep the patient intubated, and transfer them to the paediatric intensive care unit (PICU) for close monitoring.
   (d) Interventional embolization: Consider interventional embolization if conventional methods fail to control the bleeding.
   (e) Ligation of the external carotid artery: In severe and unmanageable cases, ligation of the external carotid artery may be necessary to control the haemorrhage.

7. **What is the blood supply of the tonsil?**
   Arterial:
   - Superior:
     – Tonsillar branch of the ascending pharyngeal artery
     – Lesser (descending) palatine artery (a branch of the maxillary artery of the external carotid artery)
   - Middle:
     – Tonsillar branch of the facial artery (a branch of the external carotid artery)
   - Inferior:
     – Two dorsal lingual arteries (branches of the lingual artery of the external carotid artery)
     – Ascending palatine artery
   Venous:
   - Peritonsillar vein, draining into the pharyngeal and lingual plexus, which ultimately drains into the internal jugular vein (IJV)
8. **Name common instruments used in cold dissection tonsillectomy:**
   - Draffin rods
   - Boyle-Davis mouth gag
   - Dennis Brown tonsil-holding forceps
   - Negus artery forceps
   - Negus knot pusher
   - Birkett straight forceps
   - Gwynne Evans dissector
   - Mollison retractor

5.3 Subglottic Stenosis Repair

Indications for Surgery [3]

- Subglottic stenosis causing significant airway obstruction
- Persistent or recurrent symptoms despite conservative management
- Difficulty in weaning from tracheostomy or intubation

Specific Risks Involved with the Surgery [3]

- Recurrence of stenosis
- Incomplete improvement in airway patency
- Airway oedema or granulation tissue formation
- Injury to recurrent laryngeal nerves
- Voice changes

Steps of the Surgery

1. Anaesthesia: Administer general anaesthesia, and provide appropriate airway management.
2. Positioning: Place the patient in the supine position with a head ring and shoulder bolster to extend the neck to expose the laryngeal region.
3. Perform a microlaryngoscopy and bronchoscopy (using an endoscope or microscope) to visualize the subglottic region and assess the extent and severity of the stenosis using endotracheal sizing/Myer-Cotton grading.
4. If a mild subglottis stenosis is identified: **endoscopic balloon dilatation or cold steel incisions with or without steroid injection**.
5. If a severe stenosis is identified: **tracheostomy, laryngotracheal reconstruction, or cricotracheal resection is considered**.
6. **Laryngotracheal reconstruction:** Following an MLB for measurements and planning, the airway is reconstructed using autologous tissue grafts, rib costal cartilage grafts, or other suitable materials to formulate an anterior graft, posterior graft, or both anterior and posterior grafts to widen the subglottic airway.
7. Repair is either taken as a **single-stage procedure** (more often in grade 1–2 subglottic stenosis; this is where the patient remains intubated on the paediatric intensive care unit to allow the graft to heal and is then extubated a few days later) or as a **two-stage procedure** (often in grade 3–4 stenosis, or patients with a tracheostomy in situ/other comorbidities that may make a single-stage procedure less appropriate, e.g. syndromes/significant neurological issues).
8. Cricotracheal resection: Following an MLB, the stenotic segment is resected via an open approach and anastomosis of the trachea with PDS and Vicryl sutures. The patient is kept intubated, downsized, and extubated a few days later.
9. Closure: Close any incisions using sutures, and place a temporary tracheostomy tube if required to ensure adequate post-operative airway patency.
10. Post-operative care: Monitor the patient for any complications, such as airway oedema, infection, pneumothorax, or bleeding, and provide appropriate treatment as needed. Single-stage procedures are kept on PICU, whereas two-stage procedures with a tracheostomy can return to the ward usually. A repeat airway endoscopy is carried out at intervals to assess the airway and remove any granulation tissue and any subsequent airway expansion approaches (e.g. balloon dilatation) as required.

Important Points to Note During the Surgery

- Proper assessment of the severity and extent of the subglottic stenosis is crucial for selecting the appropriate surgical technique.
- Minimizing trauma to the surrounding structures, particularly the recurrent laryngeal nerves, is essential to reduce the risk of complications.
- Meticulous airway reconstruction is required to optimize post-operative airway patency and minimize the risk of restenosis.

Questions a Consultant Might Ask a Trainee About the Operation

1. **What are the common aetiologies of subglottic stenosis?**
   Common aetiologies of subglottic stenosis are either acquired, congenital, or idiopathic. Acquired includes prolonged intubation or tracheostomy, laryngotracheal trauma, autoimmune diseases, and infections. Congenital could be cartilaginous or membranous. Syndromes that increase the risk of SGS include trisomy 21, 22q11 deletion syndromes, and CHARGE.
2. **How do you differentiate between different grades of subglottic stenosis?**
   Subglottic stenosis can be classified into four grades based on the degree of airway narrowing Myer-Cotton grading system: grade I (stenosis <50%), grade II (stenosis 51–70%), grade III (stenosis 71–99%), and grade IV (complete obstruction).

   McCaffrey grading system for length of stenosis:
   - Stage I: confined to subglottis or trachea >1 cm. Stage II: Isolated subglottic >1 cm. Stage III: Subglottic and trachea not involving the glottis. Stage IV: Subglottic/trachea involving the glottis.
3. **What are the key considerations when choosing the appropriate surgical technique for subglottic stenosis repair?**
   Key considerations include the grade and extent of stenosis, the underlying aetiology, the patient's overall health and comorbidities, and the surgeon's experience and preference. Usually for grade I/II: endoscopic dilatation, e.g. balloon +/− cold steel. More complex surgical intervention is required with grade III/IV stenosis.
4. **How do you evaluate the success of subglottic stenosis repair?**
   - The success of subglottic stenosis repair is evaluated by assessing several key factors:
   - Post-operative improvement in airway patency: This is determined by measuring the diameter of the airway post-surgery and comparing it to preoperative measurements. Improved airway patency indicates a successful dilation or reconstruction of the subglottic region.
   - Symptom relief: Assessing the patient's symptoms, such as difficulty breathing (dyspnoea), stridor, and exercise tolerance, provides insight into the effectiveness of the repair. Significant symptom relief post-operatively is a positive indicator.
   - Absence of complications: Monitoring for complications such as recurrent stenosis, infection, or airway obstruction is crucial. A lack of these complications suggests a successful repair.
   - Voice and swallow outcomes: Collaboration with a speech and language therapist to evaluate the patient's voice quality and swallowing function is important. Improvement in these areas supports the overall success of the repair.
   - Objective measurements: Objective measurements like spirometry and flow-volume loops can be used to quantify improvements in airflow and respiratory function.
   Physics Behind Airway Patency: Poiseuille's Law

Poiseuille's law describes the flow of a fluid through a cylindrical tube and is highly relevant to understanding airflow through the subglottic region:

$$Q = \frac{\Delta P \cdot \pi \cdot r^4}{8 \cdot \mu \cdot L}$$

where:
- Q is the volumetric flow rate of the fluid (air in this case).
- ΔP is the pressure difference between the ends of the tube.
- r is the radius of the tube (airway).
- μ is the dynamic viscosity of the fluid.
- L is the length of the tube.

According to Poiseuille's law, the flow rate through the airway is directly proportional to the fourth power of the radius. This implies that even a small increase in the radius of the airway results in a significant increase in airflow. Therefore, successful subglottic stenosis repair, which increases the airway diameter, leads to a substantial improvement in airflow and respiratory function.

5. **What is the difference between laryngotracheal reconstruction and resection anastomosis?**

    Laryngotracheal reconstruction (LTR):
- Technique: Utilizes expansion cartilage grafting, which can be placed anteriorly, posteriorly, or both.
- Purpose: Widens the airway by augmenting the stenotic segment without removing it.
- Indications: Suitable for long-segment stenosis or cases where preserving tracheal tissue is necessary.
- Procedure: Cartilage grafts, often harvested from the ribs, are inserted to expand the narrowed section, improving airway diameter.

    Cricotracheal resection and anastomosis (CTR):
- Technique: Involves the complete excision of the stenotic segment followed by anastomosis of the proximal and distal tracheal ends.
- Purpose: Removes the diseased segment to create a direct connection between healthy tracheal segments.
- Indications: Ideal for short-segment stenosis or when the stenotic segment is irreparably damaged.
- Procedure: The stenotic section is surgically removed, and the remaining healthy tracheal ends are sutured together to restore airway patency.

    These techniques differ primarily in their approach to treating stenosis: LTR augments the existing trachea with grafts, while CTR removes the stenotic segment and reconnects the tracheal ends.

5.4 Excision of Congenital Neck Masses (Lymphatic Malformation, Thyroglossal Cyst)

Lymphatic Malformations

- These can be divided into macrocystic (cysts >2 mm in size), microcystic (cysts <2 mm in size), or mixed lymphatic malformations.
- These can be managed conservatively, with sclerotherapy or surgery.
- Surgery is in the form of excising or debulking the lymphatic malformation. Children with large microcystic/mixed malformations also have macroglossia with microcysts on the tongue (microcysts can be treated with surgery, e.g. radiofrequency ablation (coblation)). Tongue reduction can also be performed in children to help the macroglossia.

Indications for Surgery [4]

- Alternative option to sclerotherapy or where sclerotherapy has not shrunk the malformation adequately
- Symptomatic lymphatic malformation causing pain, infection, or compression of surrounding structures
- Cosmetic concerns

Specific Risks Involved with the Surgery [4]

- Recurrence of the mass
- Damage to surrounding structures, including nerves and vessels
- Infection or haematoma
- Scarring or cosmetic deformity

5.4.1 Excision of Lymphatic Malformation

Preoperative Preparation

- Obtain informed consent after discussing the potential risks and benefits of the procedure.
- Review preoperative imaging (ultrasound, CT, MRI) to delineate the extent of the lymphatic malformation.
- Ensure that necessary blood products and equipment are available.
- Administer preoperative antibiotics as prophylaxis against infection.

Surgical Steps

1. Anaesthesia: general anaesthesia with intubation, providing muscle relaxation to facilitate easy surgical access.
2. Positioning: Position the patient supine with a head ring and shoulder bolster for slight extension of the neck.
3. Ensure that the entire neck area is accessible and that the patient is stable and secure on the operating table.
4. Perform time-out to verify patient identity, surgical site, and procedure.
5. Prep and drape the neck area in a sterile fashion.
6. Mark the incision line over the mass considering cosmetic outcome, preferably along a skin crease.
7. Administer local anaesthesia with epinephrine along the marked incision line to minimize intraoperative bleeding.
8. Make a careful incision with a scalpel through the skin and subcutaneous tissues to expose the underlying mass.
9. Create skin flaps using sharp and blunt dissection to adequately expose the lymphatic malformation.
10. Initiate dissection of the lymphatic malformation from the surrounding tissue with careful attention to avoid rupture of the cyst.
11. Isolate and protect vital structures such as nerves and vessels encountered during dissection.
12. Utilize magnification and proper lighting to identify tissue planes and structures accurately (this includes cranial nerves XI and XII, marginal mandibular branch of facial nerve).
13. Employ meticulous sharp and blunt dissection to remove the lymphatic malformation in its entirety, ensuring that no locules are left behind.
14. Use bipolar cautery for haemostasis during the dissection to control bleeding.
15. If the lymphatic malformation is large or multiloculated, consider piecemeal removal while ensuring complete excision.
16. Once the lymphatic malformation is fully excised, achieve haemostasis using electrocautery and ligate larger vessels with absorbable sutures if necessary.
17. Inspect the surgical bed for any residual cystic tissue, and ensure complete removal.
18. If a drain is required, place a closed suction drain in the surgical bed.
19. Begin layered closure of the deep tissue with absorbable sutures to reapproximate the soft tissue.
20. Close the skin using subcuticular sutures or skin adhesive for optimal cosmetic results.
21. Dress the wound with sterile, non-adherent gauze followed by a gentle compression dressing.

5.4.2 Thyroglossal Duct Anomalies (Cyst/Tract)

Indications for Surgery

- Symptomatic thyroglossal duct cyst causing pain, recurrent infection, or compression of surrounding structures.
- Large cyst causing cosmetic concern.
- Rarely, the cyst can contain a thyroid malignancy.

Specific Risks Involved with the Surgery

- Recurrence of the mass
- Damage to the hypoglossal nerve, breach of the pharynx
- Infection or haematoma
- Scarring or cosmetic deformity
- Injury to the hyoid bone or thyrohyoid membrane
- **Preoperative preparation:**
  - Obtain informed consent after discussing the potential risks and benefits of the procedure.
  - Review preoperative imaging (US neck) to confirm the presence of normal thyroid gland.

Surgical Steps (1–8 as Above)

1. Linear incision or elliptical incision to incorporate infected skin/tissue.
2. Carefully dissect around infected tissue or cyst, and identify the extent of tract (can extend to thyroid isthmus).
3. Identify strap muscles, and incorporate the rim of strap muscles into dissection as a wide local excision.
4. Identify and skeletonise the hyoid bone, and cut the central portion of hyoid bone to incorporate into the specimen. Care must be taken to avoid an inadvertent pharyngotomy and to avoid damaging the hypoglossal nerve (which sits in the lateral parts of the hyoid bone). View Fig. 1.14 in Chap. 1 for visualization.
5. Identify the base of the tongue mucosa, and carefully dissect the core of base of tongue taking care to identify any tract that extends within this.
6. Once the specimen has been removed, a Valsalva manoeuvre is performed to identify any bleeding points or leak (if a pharyngotomy or defect into the tongue base is identified, this must be repaired).
7. A suction drain is usually inserted.
8. Closure is in layers (strap muscles, platysma, and skin).
9. A dressing is usually applied over the wound.

Post-operative Care

- Monitor for bleeding and neck swelling, and assess eating and drinking. Drain output is monitored, and this is usually removed 24 h after surgery.

Questions a Consultant Might Ask a Trainee About the Operation

1. **What are the common presenting symptoms of lymphatic malformation and thyroglossal duct cyst?**
    Common presenting symptoms include a painless, smooth, and fluctuant mass in the neck. In some cases, the mass may cause pain, infection, or compression of surrounding structures.
2. **What are the key imaging studies for evaluating congenital neck masses?**
    Key imaging studies include ultrasound, computed tomography (CT), and magnetic resonance imaging (MRI) to assess the size, location, and extent of the mass, as well as its relationship to surrounding structures.
3. **Why is the modified Sistrunk procedure recommended for the excision of thyroglossal duct cysts?**
    The modified Sistrunk procedure is recommended because it involves the complete removal of the thyroglossal duct cyst along with a portion of the hyoid bone and a cuff of the base of tongue, which reduces the risk of recurrence.
4. **What investigations are required prior to thyroglossal duct cyst (TGDC) surgery?**
    Ultrasound is needed to make sure that there is thyroid gland in situ and TGDC is not the only functioning thyroid tissue. Thyroid function test is also required. Some surgeons prefer to do an MRI scan of the neck for better outlining of the lesion preoperatively.
5. **Should you excise all TGDC?**
    If there is a normal-functioning thyroid gland, then yes, it is generally recommended to excise thyroglossal duct cysts (TGDCs) in children. There are several reasons for this:
    - Risk of malignancy: Although rare, there is a small risk of malignancy developing within a TGDC. Early removal mitigates this risk. There is a 1% chance of malignancy, most commonly papillary thyroid carcinoma.
    - Risk of infection: TGDCs can become infected, leading to recurrent infections and abscess formation, which can be particularly troublesome in children.
    - Symptom relief: Children with TGDCs may experience symptoms such as swelling, discomfort, and difficulty swallowing or breathing. Surgical excision can alleviate these symptoms.
    - Prevention of recurrence: The Sistrunk procedure, which involves the removal of the cyst, the tract, and part of the hyoid bone, significantly reduces the risk of recurrence.

    Research indicates that while TGDCs can sometimes be managed conservatively, the potential for complications generally makes surgical excision the preferred approach, especially in paediatric patients. It is not something that must be done immediately, but the conversation should be had; it is advised to wait until the child is at least 2 years old.

6. **What is the embryological origin of TGDC?**

    The thyroglossal duct cyst (TGDC) originates from the foramen cecum at the junction of the anterior two-thirds of the tongue base (tuberculum impar) and the posterior one-third (copula). During the seventh week of gestation, the thyroid gland descends from the foramen cecum to its final position in the neck. This descent is completed between the seventh and tenth weeks of gestation. Normally, the thyroglossal duct involutes and disappears after the thyroid has descended. However, failure of this involution results in the formation of a TGDC.

7. **What is the best management of acutely infected TGDC?**

    The best management of an acutely infected thyroglossal duct cyst includes the following steps:
    - Antibiotic therapy: Administer appropriate antibiotics to treat the infection.
    - Aspiration: If there is a collection of pus, perform needle aspiration to relieve symptoms and reduce infection.
    - Avoid incision and drainage: Incision and drainage should be avoided as much as possible because it can transform the cyst into a fistula and increase the incidence of scarring, which may interfere with subsequent definitive surgery and increase the risk of recurrence.

    The goal is to manage the acute infection conservatively to allow for a planned surgical excision (typically the modified Sistrunk procedure) once the infection has resolved, ensuring a more effective and safer removal of the TGDC.

5.5 Excision of Branchial Cleft Anomalies

Branchial cleft anomalies are developmental defects that occur due to the incomplete obliteration of the branchial apparatus during embryogenesis. They can present as cysts, sinuses, or fistulas and are classified based on their origin from the embryonic branchial clefts. Surgical intervention is often required to prevent recurrent infection, alleviate symptoms, and eliminate the risk of potential complications [5].

Branchial cleft anomalies are classified into four types based on their embryological origin and anatomical location (Table 5.1). Surgical approach and precautions vary significantly among them due to their distinct locations and relationships with critical structures. View Fig. 1.13 in Chap. 1 for visualization of different branchial cleft cysts. A cleft anomaly opens up into the skin (first and second), and a pouch anomaly typically into the pyriform fossa. Therefore, the third and fourth anomalies are pouch anomalies.

Indications for Surgery [5]

- Recurrent infection: Chronic or recurrent infections within the anomaly
- Cosmetic concerns: Visible neck mass causing aesthetic issues
- Functional impairment: Dysphagia, dyspnoea, or discomfort

Table 5.1 Classification of branchial cleft anomalies

Type	Anatomical location and features	Surgical considerations
First branchial cleft anomalies	Located near the external auditory canal and parotid gland. May require removal of tragal cartilage to prevent recurrence	**Preservation of the facial nerve** is paramount. Complete excision may involve dissection within the parotid gland
Second branchial cleft anomalies	Found along the anterior border of the sternocleidomastoid muscle, extending towards the pharynx. The most common type	**Surgical excision** involves careful identification and preservation of the carotid artery, internal jugular vein, and glossopharyngeal, vagus, and accessory nerves
Third branchial pouch anomalies	Typically present in the lower neck, potentially involving the thyroid gland and tracking up towards the pharynx	**Thyroid gland involvement** requires careful dissection to preserve thyroid function and avoid damage to the recurrent laryngeal nerve
Fourth branchial pouch anomalies	Rare, can track from the thyroid gland down to the mediastinum	**Requires comprehensive surgical planning** due to the risk of mediastinal involvement and potential impact on the parathyroid glands and recurrent laryngeal nerve

- Potential malignancy: Suspicion of neoplastic transformation

Specific Risks Involved with the Surgery [5]

- Nerve damage: Risk to the facial nerve, accessory nerve, and hypoglossal nerve
- Scarring: Potential for visible neck scarring
- Infection: Post-operative wound infection
- Haemorrhage: Risk of bleeding during and after surgery
- Recurrence: Incomplete removal leading to recurrence

Preoperative Preparation

- Thoroughly review imaging studies (ultrasound, CT, or MRI) to delineate the course of the tract, cyst size, and its relationship to key anatomical structures.
- Set up for general anaesthesia with careful positioning of the patient, ensuring neck extension for optimal surgical access as previously discussed.

Surgical Steps: Excision of a Second Branchial Cleft Anomaly

1. Make a transverse cervical incision overlying the most prominent part of the mass or the sinus opening—if a fistula is present, then perform an elliptical incision around the fistulating skin.
2. Gently dissect through subcutaneous tissue and platysma muscle to expose the deeper cervical fascia.

3. Carefully identify the cyst or sinus tract. Use blunt dissection to separate it from surrounding tissues.
4. In cases of a sinus, trace the tract towards its internal opening, which often leads towards the tonsillar fossa.
5. If the tract extends towards the pharynx, additional exposure may be required for complete excision.
6. Dissect and follow the tract carefully to avoid injury to nearby structures.
7. Dissect around the cyst or tract, maintaining a plane close to the lesion to avoid damage to adjacent structures.
8. Complete excision of the cyst or tract is essential to prevent recurrence.
9. Constant vigilance to avoid injury to the facial nerve, hypoglossal nerve, and other nearby structures.
10. Use of nerve monitoring may be beneficial, especially in complicated or recurrent cases.
11. Careful inspection and control of bleeding points using electrocautery or ligatures.
12. Ensure adequate homeostasis before closure to prevent post-operative haematoma.
13. Layered closure of the wound, including the platysma and subcutaneous tissues, to optimize cosmetic outcome.
14. Skin closure with monofilament sutures or skin adhesive for minimal scarring.
15. Monitor for immediate post-operative complications like bleeding, infection, or swelling.
16. Plan for follow-up to assess wound healing and to monitor for signs of recurrence.

Questions a Consultant Might Ask a Trainee About the Operation

1. **How does the embryological origin of branchial cleft anomalies influence their surgical management?**

   The embryological origin determines the anomaly's location and its proximity to critical structures, guiding the surgical approach. For instance, first branchial cleft anomalies, derived from the first cleft, are closely associated with the facial nerve, necessitating careful dissection to avoid nerve injury. Second branchial cleft anomalies, originating from the second cleft, lie near the sternocleidomastoid and require attention to protect the carotid artery and internal jugular vein. Surgical management of a third or fourth branchial pouch anomaly is typically endoscopic, set up similar to a microlaryngoscopy. The opening is found in the pyriform sinus and it is cauterised. Occasionally an open approach is required.

2. **What are the critical steps in ensuring complete removal of a second branchial cleft cyst to minimize recurrence, and how does its location affect these steps?**

   Complete removal involves identifying the cyst's entire tract, which may extend towards the pharyngeal wall. The cyst's location along the anterior border of the sternocleidomastoid muscle necessitates careful dissection to avoid nerve and vascular structures. Ensuring that no remnants are left behind involves

meticulous exploration of the tract and possible exposure and dissection around the carotid sheath.
3. **Describe the significance of tragal cartilage removal in the surgical excision of first branchial cleft anomalies and the rationale behind it.**
   Tragal cartilage removal is crucial for first branchial cleft anomalies that extend near the external auditory canal and may involve the parotid gland. Removing a portion of the tragal cartilage ensures complete excision of the cyst or fistula tract, reducing the risk of recurrence by eliminating potential residual epithelial tissue embedded within or adjacent to the cartilage.
4. **In the context of branchial cleft anomalies, how does the preservation of the facial nerve influence the surgical outcome, especially for anomalies close to the parotid gland?**
   Facial nerve preservation is paramount to prevent facial paralysis, affecting facial expression and function. Anomalies near the parotid gland, especially first branchial cleft anomalies, require precise dissection and often intraoperative nerve monitoring to avoid nerve damage, ensuring that the patient's facial function remains intact post-surgery.
5. **How do the potential complications of branchial cleft anomaly surgery, such as injury to major vessels or nerves, dictate the preoperative planning and intraoperative strategy?**
   Preoperative imaging like MRI or CT scans is essential to map the anomaly's relationship with vital structures, allowing for strategic surgical planning. Intraoperatively, techniques such as nerve monitoring and careful dissection are employed to identify and preserve these structures, minimizing the risk of complications like haemorrhage or nerve injury.

References

1. Randall DA. Current indications for tonsillectomy and adenoidectomy. J Am Board Fam Med. 2020;33(6):1025–30.
2. National Institute for Health and Care Excellence (NICE). Otitis media with effusion in under 12s. NICE guideline [NG233]. 2023 Aug 30. Available from: https://www.nice.org.uk/guidance/ng233
3. Jefferson ND, Cohen AP, Rutter MJ. Subglottic stenosis. Semin Pediatr Surg. 2016;25(3):138–43.
4. Erikci V, Hoşgör M. Management of congenital neck lesions in children. J Plast Reconstr Aesthet Surg. 2014;67(9):e217–22.
5. Zaifullah S, Yunus MR, See GB. Diagnosis and treatment of branchial cleft anomalies in UKMMC: a 10-year retrospective study. Eur Arch Otorrinolaringol. 2013;270:1501–6.

Emergencies

Sameer Mallick, Zohaib Siddiqui, Basim Wahba, and Keli Dusu

6.1 Emergency Tracheostomy (Including under Local Anaesthetic)

Cannot intubate, can ventilate.

Indications for Surgery [1]

- Acute airway obstruction (e.g. foreign body, tumour, angioedema)
- Failed endotracheal intubation
- Severe facial trauma obstructing the airway
- Severe laryngeal trauma
- Upper airway burns with impending airway compromise

Specific Risks Involved with the Surgery [1]

- Bleeding
- Infection
- Damage to surrounding structures (e.g. nerves, vessels, oesophagus)

S. Mallick (✉)
Nottingham University Hospital, Nottingham, Nottinghamshire, UK
e-mail: s.mallick1@nhs.net

Z. Siddiqui
Medway NHS Foundation Trust, Gillingham, Kent, UK

B. Wahba
Queen Victoria Hospital, East Grinstead, West Sussex, UK

K. Dusu
Frimley Park Hospital, Frimley, Camberley, UK

© The Author(s), under exclusive license to Springer Nature Switzerland AG 2024
Z. Siddiqui et al. (eds.), *Essentials of ENT Surgical Procedures*,
https://doi.org/10.1007/978-3-031-71394-1_6

- Pneumothorax or pneumomediastinum
- Subcutaneous emphysema
- Tracheal stenosis
- False passage creation

Steps of the Surgery

1. Ensure that you have the correct tracheostomy tube for your patient and a size up and down to be safe. Check the cuff inflates of the tube you would like to use. If the patient has a large amount of subcutaneous fascia, you may require an adjustable flange tube.
2. Position the patient supine with a head ring and shoulder roll for neck extension.
3. Identify, palpate, and mark the cricoid cartilage, thyroid cartilage, and sternal notch.
4. Administer local anaesthesia by injecting lidocaine with epinephrine into the skin and subcutaneous tissues over the planned incision site. You can also carefully inject deeper down towards trachea.
5. Make a horizontal (or vertical) skin incision approximately 2–3 cm in length between the cricoid cartilage and the sternal notch. If required, increase the incision size for access.
6. Dissect through the subcutaneous tissue, midline dissection through strap muscles, and pre-tracheal fascia using a combination of blunt dissection, a haemostat, and scissors (depends on preference).
7. If thyroid isthmus is visualized (usually inferior to cricoid), ligate or carefully dissect through this. If left alone in close proximity to the tracheostomy, it may bleed due to the tube rubbing against it. If retracted only, and the tube is dislodged, the isthmus may cover your tracheostomy incision.
8. Identification of trachea: Carefully identify the trachea between the second and fourth tracheal rings. You can aim to identify cricoid first and work down.
9. Tracheal incision: Make a vertical incision between the second and fourth tracheal rings using a scalpel (11 blade) as seen in Fig. 6.1. If you expect subglottic cancer, consider high tracheostomy. Alternatively, a tracheal window or a "U"-shaped incision can be made, with the base of the "U" being at the inferior aspect of the tracheal ring (Bjork flap). During the incision, make sure that your surgical team and anaesthetic team are aware. You will need your colleague to apply suction at this point to prevent blood from entering the trachea and to suction secretions from the trachea as the patient will likely cough.
10. Tracheal dilatation: Dilate the tracheal incision using a curved haemostat or tracheal dilator if required.
11. Tube insertion: Insert the tracheostomy tube (apply lubrication to the tube prior) through the tracheal incision, directing it caudally towards the carina. Inflate the cuff, and confirm proper placement by checking CO_2 trace, auscultating for bilateral breath sounds and observing for adequate chest rise.

Fig. 6.1 Tracheostomy incision and insertion. Illustrated by Vikum Liyanaarachchi

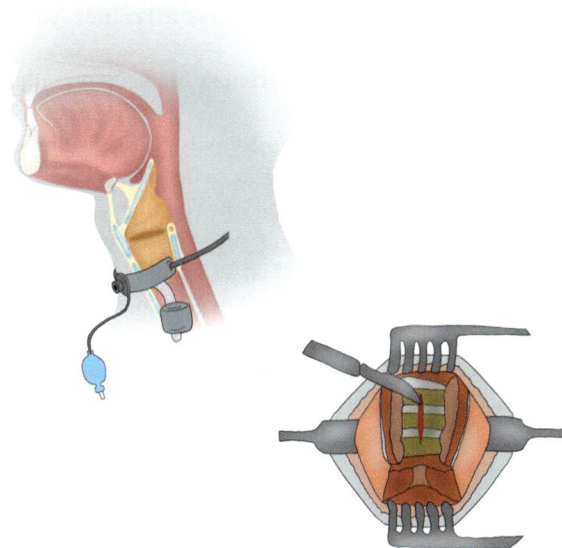

(a) If the patient was under general anaesthetic, once the incision was made, you would ask the team to start slowly removing the ET tube; once it has passed your tracheal incision, you may insert your tracheostomy tube and place the GA through it.
12. Secure the tube: Secure the tracheostomy tube with sutures and a tracheostomy tie or other suitable fixation devices.
13. Monitor the patient: Monitor the patient for any complications, and provide appropriate post-operative care.

Important Points to Note During the Surgery

- In an emergency setting, speed and accuracy are crucial for the success of the procedure.
- Adequate local anaesthesia is important for patient comfort and to minimize complications, but be prepared for the possibility of needing to convert to general anaesthesia if required.
- Careful dissection and identification of the trachea can help minimize injury to surrounding structures.
- Proper placement of the tracheostomy tube and securing it in place are essential to maintain the patient's airway.

Questions a Consultant Might Ask a Trainee About the Operation

1. **What are the main differences between an emergency tracheostomy and an elective tracheostomy?**
   An emergency tracheostomy is performed in an urgent setting with an immediate need for airway access, whereas an elective tracheostomy is planned and performed in a controlled environment. An emergency tracheostomy may be performed under local anaesthesia, whereas an elective tracheostomy is typically performed under general anaesthesia [1].
2. **Why would the operating surgeon divide the thyroid isthmus?**
   If the thyroid isthmus is obstructing your view of the tracheal rings, the options are to either divide it for access or retract it. If retracted and tracheostomy is placed, the thyroid isthmus can rub on the tracheostomy tube which can lead to bleeding. Also, if the patient is decannulated accidentally in the immediate post-operative period, it might be more challenging to get the tube back into position as the isthmus may now cover the tracheostomy incision.
3. **What are the potential complications of a tracheostomy performed under local anaesthesia?**
   Potential complications include inadequate anaesthesia leading to patient discomfort and movement, difficulty maintaining the airway, and an increased risk of injury to surrounding structures due to patient movement [1]. In some cases, conversion to general anaesthesia may be necessary.
4. **How can you confirm correct placement of the tracheostomy tube?**
   Correct placement of the tracheostomy tube can be confirmed by auscultating for bilateral breath sounds, observing for adequate chest rise, and monitoring the patient's oxygen saturation and end-tidal CO_2 levels. The National Confidential Enquiry into Patient Outcome and Death (NCEPOD) mentions that a fibre-optic bronchoscope should be used to visualize the tracheostomy tube's position within the trachea.
5. **What guidelines do you know regarding emergency tracheostomy protocols?**
   National Tracheostomy Safety Project (NTSP) [2]
   Difficult Airway Society (DAS) Difficult Intubation Protocol Guidelines 2015 [3]
6. **What post-operative instructions do you need to give to the ward?**
   - The cuff should not be overinflated, to prevent ischaemic damage to the tracheal wall. Use a pressure gauge to check the cuff's pressure (should be between 20 and 25 mmHg). Release the pressure in the cuff after 24 h, unless the patient is being ventilated.
   - Patient must be given humidification for at least the first 48 h to reduce tracheal crusting.
   - Regular suctioning of the airway to clear secretions may be needed.
   - A spare tracheostomy tube (and smaller sizes), an introducer, and tracheal dilators should be kept by the patient's bed in case of accidental displacement of the tube.
   - The first tube change should take place after about 5–7 days, when a track is well formed.

7. **What are the differences in an emergency tracheostomy performed in children?**
   - In children, the trachea is a thin and very malleable structure. It may require stabilization when handling. If uncertain, you can check the location by inserting a needle to make sure that air bubbles are seen in saline-filled syringe. Avoid too much lateral dissection (to avoid injury to lateral structures) and inferior dissection (pleura is relatively high).
   - Slit tracheal incision—no window or Bjork flap.
   - Vicryl stomal maturation suture and Prolene stay sutures.
8. **What is the protocol for adult tracheostomy decannulation?**
   - Cuff deflation.
   - Progressive deflation: Consider downsizing and/or fenestrated tube and/or cuffless tube.
   - Capping off the tracheostomy tube with progressive length during the day and then overnight with one-to-one nurse observation.
   - Decannulation.

6.2 Cricothyroidotomy

Indications for Surgery [4]

- Acute airway obstruction (e.g. foreign body, laryngeal oedema, tumour)
- Failed endotracheal intubation—*cannot intubate, cannot ventilate*
- Severe facial trauma obstructing the airway
- Severe laryngeal trauma
- Immediate need for a secure airway in a life-threatening situation

Specific Risks Involved with the Surgery [4]

- Bleeding
- Infection
- Damage to surrounding structures (e.g. nerves, vessels, larynx)
- Subcutaneous emphysema
- Tracheal stenosis
- Tracheo-oesophageal fistula
- False passage creation

Steps of the Surgery (Scalpel, Bougie, Tube)

1. Patient preparation: Position the patient supine with the neck extended, if possible. This position provides better access to the neck and airway.
2. Palpation: Quickly identify the cricoid cartilage and the cricothyroid membrane, which is located between the cricoid and thyroid cartilages.

3. Local anaesthesia (if applicable): If time and patient condition permit, inject local anaesthesia (like lidocaine) into the skin over the cricothyroid membrane. In many emergency situations, there might not be enough time for this step.
4. Skin incision: Make a small vertical skin incision of about 3–5 cm, then identify cricothyroid membrane, and then make a horizontal incision (about 2–3 cm) over the cricothyroid membrane. The incision should be swift and precise. Direct scalpel caudally to avoid the vocal cords and posterior tracheal wall injury.
5. Membrane puncture: Stabilize the larynx with one hand—also known as the "laryngeal handshake". With the other hand, use a scalpel to puncture the cricothyroid membrane in a vertical direction. This is often done in a "stab" fashion to quickly enter the airway. This can be seen in Fig. 6.2.
6. Bougie insertion (if available): If a bougie is available, insert it through the incision into the trachea to guide the tube placement.
7. Tube insertion: Insert a small endotracheal tube or a cricothyroidotomy tube over the bougie or directly through the incision into the trachea.

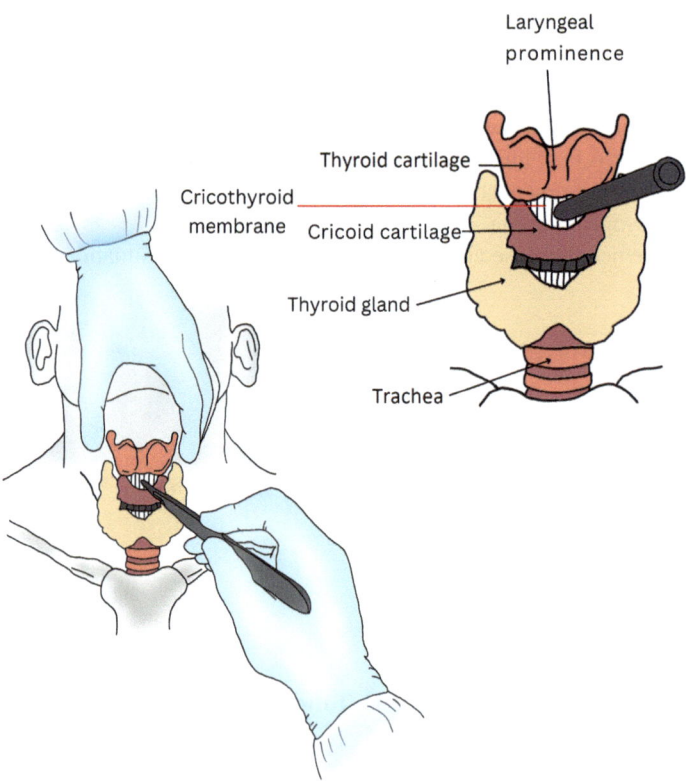

Fig. 6.2 Cricothyroidotomy with anatomy and laryngeal handshake. Illustrated by Vikum Liyanaarachchi

6 Emergencies

8. Confirm placement: Inflate the cuff of the tube, and confirm placement by end-tidal CO_2 trace, listening for breath sounds and observing chest rise. This step is critical to ensure that the tube is in the trachea and not in surrounding tissues.
9. Secure the tube: Secure the tube in place to prevent displacement. This can be done with ties or adhesive tape.
10. Monitor the patient: Continuously monitor the patient for any complications, and provide immediate post-procedure care.
11. Prepare the patient for a surgical tracheostomy as the patient's airway is still unstable.

Important Points to Note During the Surgery

- Cricothyroidotomy is a life-saving procedure and should be performed quickly and efficiently.
- Proper identification of the cricothyroid membrane is crucial for the success of the procedure.
- Proper placement of the tube and securing it in place are essential to maintain the patient's airway.
- Cricothyroidotomy is typically considered a temporary solution; definitive airway management (e.g. tracheostomy) may be needed after stabilization.
- Simplified down to scalpel, bougie, and tube.

Questions a Consultant Might Ask a Trainee About the Operation

1. **In which situations would you choose to perform a cricothyroidotomy over a tracheostomy?**
    A cricothyroidotomy is indicated in emergency situations where there is an immediate need for a secure airway, such as acute airway obstruction, failed endotracheal intubation, severe facial or laryngeal trauma, and life-threatening situations where other airway management techniques are unsuccessful or contraindicated. A tracheostomy, on the other hand, is a more controlled procedure usually performed electively or semi-electively for patients requiring long-term airway management, such as in cases of chronic airway obstruction, prolonged mechanical ventilation, or recurrent aspiration. When you have a patient who is unable to ventilate or intubate, then a cricothyroidotomy is performed. If you can ventilate (for example, with an iGel or bag-valve mask), then a surgical tracheostomy under local anaesthetic can be performed.
2. **What is the appropriate tube size for a cricothyroidotomy, and why is this important?**
    A small endotracheal tube (e.g. size 6.0) or a specific cricothyroidotomy tube is typically used for a cricothyroidotomy. Using an appropriately sized tube is important to minimize trauma to the surrounding structures, reduce the risk of complications, and ensure adequate ventilation.

3. **How can you confirm correct placement of the cricothyroidotomy tube?**
   Correct placement of the cricothyroidotomy tube can be confirmed by auscultating for bilateral breath sounds, observing for adequate chest rise, and monitoring the patient's oxygen saturation and end-tidal CO_2 levels.
4. **What are the key landmarks to identify When performing a cricothyroidotomy?**
   The key landmarks for a cricothyroidotomy are the cricoid cartilage and the cricothyroid membrane, which is located between the cricoid and thyroid cartilages. Correct identification and palpation of these landmarks are crucial for the success of the procedure [4].
5. **How can you identify the cricothyroid membrane?**
   The laryngeal handshake technique described in the DAS 2015 guidelines:
   (a) With the index finger and thumb grasp the top of the larynx (the greater cornu of the hyoid bone) and roll it from side to side.
   (b) The fingers and thumb slide down over the thyroid laminae.
   (c) Middle finger and thumb rest on the cricoid cartilage, with the index finger palpating the cricothyroid membrane.

6.3 Epistaxis Control with Sphenopalatine Artery (SPA) Ligation

Indications for Surgery [5]

- Uncontrolled anterior or posterior nasal bleeding
- Failure of conservative measures (e.g. nasal packing, chemical cautery)
- Recurrent epistaxis
- Bleeding disorders

Specific Risks Involved with the Surgery [5]

- Nasal septal perforation
- Infection
- Rebleeding
- Pain or discomfort
- Aspiration (for posterior nasal packing)
- Injury to surrounding structures during arterial ligation

Steps of the Surgery (Sphenopalatine Artery (SPA) Ligation)

1. Preparation: Administer general anaesthesia, and position the patient supine with the head slightly extended with reversed Trendelenburg position. This position provides optimal access to the nasal cavity.
2. Decongestion: Apply a topical decongestant (like xylometazoline, adrenaline, or Moffett's solution) to the nasal cavity. This helps reduce mucosal oedema and improves visualization during the procedure.
3. Endoscopic examination: Perform a diagnostic nasal endoscopy to identify the source of bleeding and any underlying pathology.
4. Middle meatus exposure: Gently medialize the middle turbinate using an endoscopic suction or a Freer elevator. This step exposes the middle meatus for better access to the sphenopalatine foramen.
5. Location of incision: The incision is typically made in the lateral nasal wall, specifically in the region of the posterior aspect of the middle meatus. This area is posterior to the middle turbinate and superior to the horizontal portion of the palatine bone.
6. Making the incision: A sharp instrument, like a scalpel or a sickle knife, is used to make a vertical incision in the mucosa of the lateral nasal wall. This incision is usually about 1–1.5 cm in length.
7. Elevation of mucoperiosteal flap: Following the incision, a mucoperiosteal flap is elevated using a Freer elevator (suction Freer works well) or a similar instrument. This step is performed carefully to avoid damaging the underlying structures. Fig. 6.3 shows this.
8. Exposure of the sphenopalatine foramen: Once the mucoperiosteal flap is elevated, the underlying bone of the lateral nasal wall is exposed. The sphenopalatine foramen, a key landmark in this surgery, is in this bony area.
9. Crista ethmoidalis may be removed using a Kerrison rongeur or a high-speed drill to better expose the foramen and the SPA.

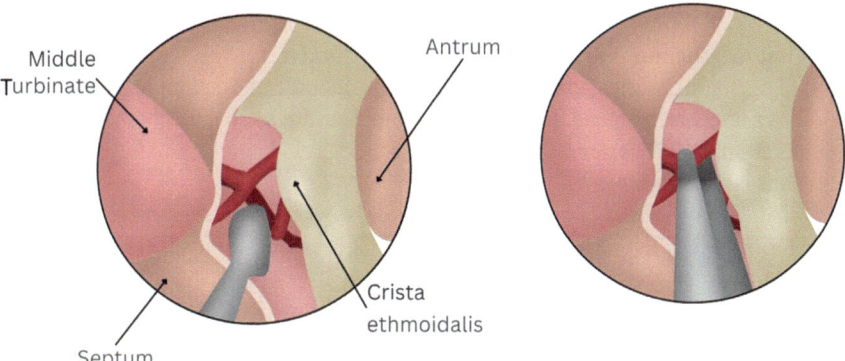

Fig. 6.3 SPA ligation with mucoperiosteal flap raised and blood vessels being cauterized with bipolar forceps. Illustrated by Vikum Liyanaarachchi

10. Identification of the sphenopalatine artery: The SPA typically emerges from the sphenopalatine foramen. At this stage, careful dissection is needed to identify the artery. Bleeding from the SPA or its branches may occur during this dissection, which helps in identifying the artery. See Fig. 6.3.
11. Inferior uncinectomy with middle meatal antrostomy could be done for better visualization and orientation and for suctioning of blood trapped in the maxillary sinus.
12. Cauterization or clipping: Ligate the sphenopalatine artery using bipolar electrocautery or endoscopic clips. The choice between cauterization and clipping may depend on the surgeon's preference and the specific clinical scenario.
13. Confirmation of haemostasis: After ligation, assess the surgical site to ensure adequate haemostasis and the absence of active bleeding.
14. Nasal packing (if necessary): If bleeding continues despite the ligation, consider placing anterior or posterior nasal packing to apply pressure and control the bleeding.
15. Post-operative care: Monitor the patient for complications, manage pain with appropriate analgesia, and schedule follow-up visits for proper healing assessment and, if used, removal of nasal packing.

Important Points to Note During the Surgery

- Adequate visualization is crucial for a successful procedure.
- Be gentle during endoscopic manipulation to minimize the risk of injury to surrounding structures.
- Ensure proper identification of the sphenopalatine artery before ligation.
- Monitor the patient closely for any signs of rebleeding or complications post-operatively.

Questions a Consultant Might Ask a Trainee About the Operation

1. **What are the main arteries involved in epistaxis?**
   The main arteries involved in epistaxis include the sphenopalatine artery (SPA), the anterior and posterior ethmoidal arteries, and the branches of the internal maxillary artery.
2. **What is Little's area?**
   Little's area, also known as Kiesselbach's plexus, is a region located in the anterior part of the nasal septum (Fig. 6.4). It is an anastomosis of five arteries:
   - Anterior ethmoidal artery
   - Posterior ethmoidal artery
   - Sphenopalatine artery
   - Greater palatine artery
   - Septal branch of the superior labial artery

   This area is highly vascularized, making it a common site for anterior nosebleeds.

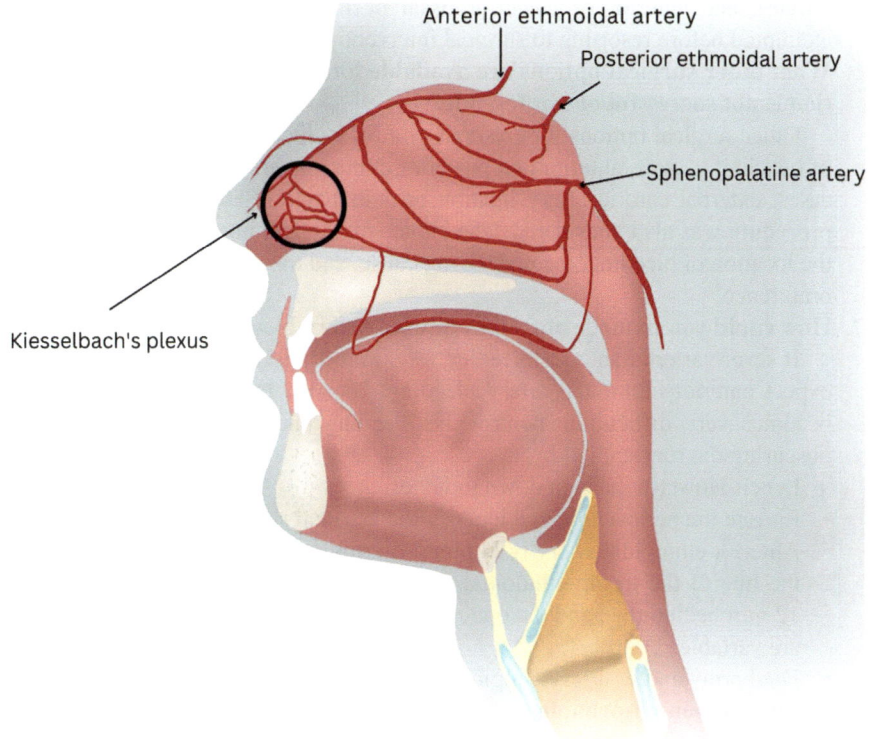

Fig. 6.4 Little's area (Kiesselbach's plexus) with its arterial supply. Illustrated by Vikum Liyanaarachchi

3. **What is the significance of the sphenopalatine artery in epistaxis management?**

    The sphenopalatine artery is a major blood supply to the nasal cavity and is often the source of posterior epistaxis. Ligation or cauterization of the SPA can effectively control bleeding in cases where conservative measures have failed.

4. **How can you differentiate between anterior and posterior epistaxis?**

    Anterior epistaxis typically presents with blood flowing from the nostril(s), while posterior epistaxis can present with blood flowing into the oropharynx, causing the patient to swallow blood and potentially leading to nausea, vomiting, or aspiration.

5. **What are the conservative measures typically employed before resorting to surgical intervention for epistaxis?**

    Conservative measures for epistaxis control include nasal compression, application of topical vasoconstrictors or decongestants, chemical cautery (e.g. silver

nitrate), and anterior or posterior nasal packing. These measures are often attempted before resorting to surgical intervention.
6. **What other surgical options are available for epistaxis control if SPA ligation is not successful or not feasible?**
   Other surgical options for epistaxis control include endoscopic cauterization of bleeding vessels, anterior and posterior ethmoidal artery ligation, and, in rare cases, external carotid artery ligation or embolization. Historically, a Young's procedure was also considered. The choice of surgical intervention depends on the location of bleeding, the underlying cause, and the surgeon's experience and preference.
7. **How could you manage anterior ethmoid artery bleeding?**
   If severe arterial anterior bleeding (e.g. immediately after FESS), one could expect anterior ethmoidal artery bleeding. Usually, the artery retracts, and it becomes very difficult to control the bleeding endoscopically due to blood obscuring the surgical field.
   Lynch-Howarth incision down to bone:
   - Elevate the periosteum, and identify the lacrimal sac.
   - Anterior ethmoidal artery is 24 mm posterior to the anterior lacrimal crest, in the line of the fronto-ethmoidal suture. The posterior ethmoidal artery lies 12 mm behind this, and the optic nerve is 6 mm behind this. These distances are variable.
   - Diathermy and/or artery clipping could be used to control bleeding.
8. **What common absorbable materials could be used to control bleeding?**
   - Floseal: bovine gelatine with human lyophilized human thrombin
   - Surgiflo: porcine gelatin with human thrombin
   - Kaltostat: alginate
   - Surgicel: cellulose
   - Tisseel as fibrin glue: human plasma cryoprecipitate

6.4 Foreign Body Removal (Ear, Nose, Throat)

Indications for Surgery

- Presence of a foreign body in the ear, nose, or throat.
- Failure of conservative measures to remove the foreign body.
- Risk of complications or injury due to the foreign body.

Specific Risks Involved with the Surgery

- Injury to surrounding structures
- Infection
- Bleeding
- Retention or migration of the foreign body

6 Emergencies   177

- Aspiration (for foreign bodies in the throat)
- Anaesthesia complications (for rigid oesophagoscopy)

Steps of the Surgery

- Preparation: Administer appropriate anaesthesia (local or general, depending on the location of the foreign body and the patient's condition).

  Ear foreign body removal techniques:

- Irrigation: Use a syringe to gently flush the ear canal with warm water, attempting to float the foreign body out.
- Suction: Apply gentle suction using a small catheter to remove the foreign body from the ear canal.
- Forceps: Carefully grasp the foreign body with forceps or crocodile forceps, and gently remove it, as seen in Fig. 6.5.
- Loop or hook: Use a small loop or hook to dislodge and remove the foreign body, as seen in Fig. 6.6.

  Nose foreign body removal techniques:

- Parent's kiss: Have the parent or caregiver close the child's mouth and deliver a short, forceful puff of air into the child's mouth, which can propel the foreign body out of the nostril.
- Positive pressure: Have the patient occlude the unaffected nostril and exhale forcefully through the affected nostril.
- Forceps or suction: Use forceps, a suction catheter, or a specialized foreign body removal instrument to gently extract the foreign body.

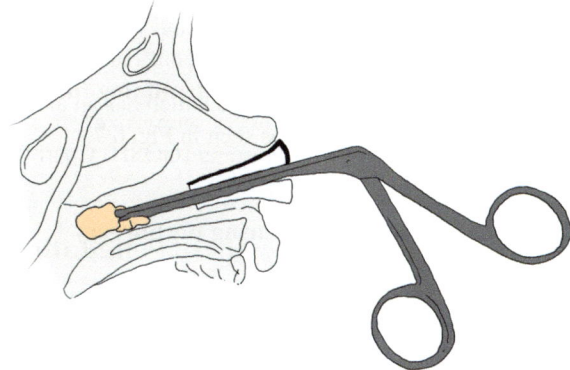

Fig. 6.5 Foreign body being removed from ear canal with crocodile forceps. Illustrated by Vikum Liyanaarachchi

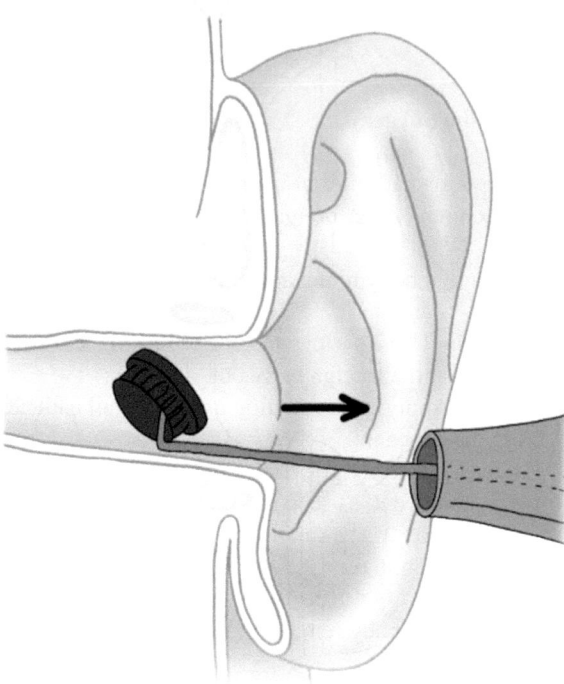

Fig. 6.6 Foreign body being removed from ear canal with wax hook. Illustrated by Vikum Liyanaarachchi

Throat foreign body removal techniques:

- Rigid oesophagoscopy: Use a rigid oesophagoscope to visualize the foreign body and extract it using forceps or other specialized instruments.
- Flexible endoscopy: In some cases, a flexible endoscope can be used to visualize and remove the foreign body.
- Surgical intervention: In rare cases, a surgical intervention may be required to remove an impacted or hazardous foreign body in the throat.

Tracheal foreign bodies:

- Use a ventilating bronchoscope which has an ability to visualize, grasp, suction, and ventilate the patient, as seen in Fig. 6.7.

Important Points to Note During the Surgery

- Adequate visualization and atraumatic techniques are essential to minimize the risk of complications.

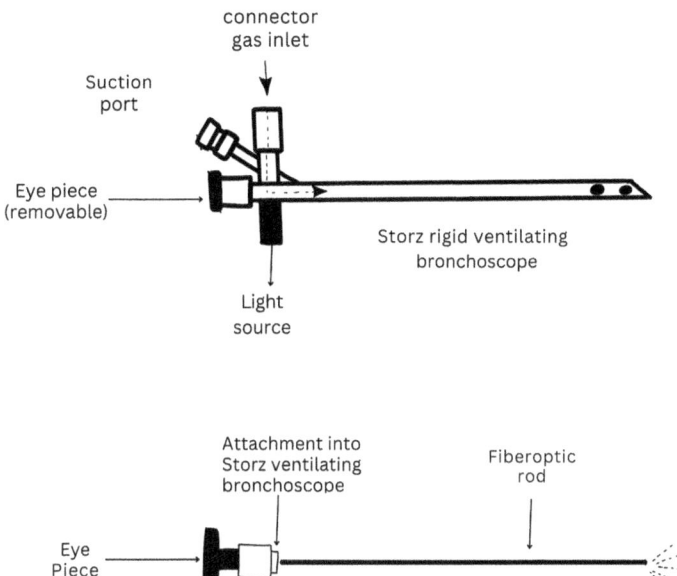

Fig. 6.7 Ventilating bronchoscope. Illustrated by Vikum Liyanaarachchi

- Be prepared to manage potential complications, such as bleeding or airway obstruction.
- Monitor the patient closely for any signs of complications or retained foreign body fragments.

Questions a Consultant Might Ask a Trainee About the Operation

1. **When should you avoid using irrigation to remove an ear foreign body?**
   Irrigation should be avoided if the foreign body is organic (e.g. seeds, insects), as water can cause the foreign body to swell or become more difficult to remove. It should also be avoided if there is a known or suspected tympanic membrane perforation.
2. **What are the potential complications of using forceps or other instruments to remove a nasal foreign body?**
   Potential complications include injury to the nasal mucosa, bleeding, or accidental pushing of the foreign body further into the nasal cavity.

3. **Why is rigid oesophagoscopy preferred over flexible endoscopy for throat foreign body removal in some cases?**

   Rigid oesophagoscopy allows for better visualization, more precise control, and use of specialized instruments for foreign body removal. It may be preferred in cases where the foreign body is large, sharp, or impacted.

4. **In which situations is surgical intervention necessary for throat foreign body removal?**

   Surgical intervention may be required for foreign bodies that cannot be safely removed using endoscopic techniques and are causing severe symptoms or complications (e.g. airway obstruction, perforation) or if the foreign body has migrated to an inaccessible location.

5. **How can you minimize the risk of aspiration during foreign body removal from the throat?**

   To minimize the risk of aspiration, ensure proper patient positioning, use adequate anaesthesia, maintain airway patency, and use atraumatic techniques during foreign body removal. Be prepared to manage airway complications if they arise and consider consultation with an anaesthesiologist or intensivist for complex cases or high-risk patients.

6. **Is it safe to wait for the next day in cases of foreign body inhalation?**

   Yes, if the foreign body has been identified and is not considered high risk such as a button battery or if the object is sharp. If the child is distressed however, then you may consider removing it sooner. It is important to recognise that this is an emergency and where possible it should be removed as soon as possible.

7. **What are the types of bronchoscopy?**
   - Flexible fibre-optic bronchoscopy.
   - Rigid:
     - Ventilating bronchoscope as seen in Fig. 6.7.
     - Venturi: The Venturi bronchoscopes are essentially open-ended metal tubes. Gas exchange is brought about by jet insufflation of the lungs with oxygen and entrained air using a Sanders injection. This technique is only used in patients >40 kg due to high risk of barotrauma.

8. **How can you identify the size of the bronchoscope?**

   In general, it is half a degree below age-appropriate ETT (ID). The correct size is the one that allows an audible leak at 20 cm H_2O pressure. One can also find the correct size (age dependant) on the appropriate chart mounted on the theatre.

6.5 Drainage of Deep Neck Infections (Peritonsillar, Parapharyngeal, Retropharyngeal Abscesses)

Indications for Surgery

- Clinical or radiological evidence of a deep neck abscess (peritonsillar, parapharyngeal, retropharyngeal)
- Failure of conservative management, such as antibiotics and observation

- Compromised airway or risk of airway compromise
- Evidence of sepsis or systemic infection

Specific Risks Involved with the Surgery

- Injury to adjacent structures (e.g. nerves, blood vessels, salivary glands)
- Incomplete drainage or recurrence of the abscess
- Aspiration
- Bleeding
- Infection
- Anaesthesia complications

Steps of the Surgery

1. Preparation: Administer appropriate anaesthesia (local or general, depending on the location of the abscess and the patient's condition), secure the airway, and position the patient.

Peritonsillar abscess drainage:

1. Identify the point of maximum fluctuance, typically above the superior pole of the tonsil.
2. Infiltrate the area with local anaesthesia and a vasoconstrictor.
3. Make a small incision at the point of maximum fluctuance, and use a blunt instrument to open up and break up loculations (Hilton method) allowing for pus drainage.
4. Gently express pus from the abscess cavity and irrigate with saline.

Parapharyngeal abscess drainage:

1. Perform a transcervical approach, making an incision along the anterior border of the sternocleidomastoid muscle or horizontal incision at the level of hyoid bone, two finger breadths below the angle of mandible.
2. Transoral approach could be considered with ipsilateral tonsillectomy if the parapharyngeal abscess is high up and close to the tonsil and lateral to superior constrictor muscle.
3. Carefully dissect through the subplatysmal and investing fascia to reach the carotid sheath.
4. Retract the carotid sheath and its contents laterally to expose the parapharyngeal space.
5. Slide a finger along the posterior belly of digastric and stylohyoid muscles to reach the styloid process in the parapharyngeal space.
6. Incise the fascia overlying the abscess and drain the pus.

7. Break up loculations and irrigate with saline.
8. Place a drain if necessary to facilitate ongoing drainage.

Retropharyngeal abscess drainage:

1. Perform a transoral or transcervical approach or both, depending on the location and size of the abscess and the patient's anatomy.
2. Transoral approach: Under direct visualization, incise the posterior pharyngeal wall at the point of maximum bulging. Drain the pus and irrigate with saline.
3. Transcervical approach: Make an incision along the anterior border of the sternocleidomastoid muscle, and dissect to reach the retropharyngeal space.
4. Locate carotid sheath:
    - Identify the sternocleidomastoid muscle; the carotid sheath is located medial to it, containing the carotid artery, internal jugular vein, and vagus nerve.
5. Identify middle thyroid vein:
    - Locate the vein as it drains from the thyroid gland into the internal jugular vein.
    - Ligate the vein early in the procedure to allow for medial mobilization of the thyroid gland, facilitating access to deeper neck structures.
6. Medialize thyroid gland:
    - Following ligation of the middle thyroid vein, carefully mobilize the thyroid gland medially.
    - This step provides the necessary space to access the deeper planes leading to the retropharyngeal space.
7. Access retropharyngeal space:
    - Continue dissection medially behind the pharynx, carefully navigating through the fascial planes.
    - The carotid sheath lies lateral to the retropharyngeal space. This means that when accessing the retropharyngeal space, the dissection is generally performed medially (towards the midline) away from the carotid sheath to prevent injury to its contents.
    - Reach the retropharyngeal space by dissecting posterior to the pharyngeal musculature.
    - Incise the fascia overlying the abscess, drain the pus, and irrigate with saline. If extended to mediastinum, the incision can be extended down to the level of T4.
8. Place a drain if necessary to facilitate ongoing drainage.

Important Points to Note During the Surgery

- Understand the relevant anatomy, including the location of major blood vessels, nerves, and other structures.
- Be prepared to manage potential complications, such as bleeding or airway compromise.
- Monitor the patient closely for any signs of complications or recurrence of infection.

Questions a Consultant Might Ask a Trainee About the Operation

1. **What are the boundaries of the parapharyngeal space?**
   The parapharyngeal space is bordered by the skull base superiorly; the hyoid bone inferiorly; the parotid gland, digastric, and lateral pterygoid laterally; the superior constrictor medially; retropharyngeal space posteromedially; and carotid sheath posterolaterally. It is bounded anteriorly by pterygomandibular raphe. It is divided into anterior (prestyloid) and posterior (poststyloid) compartments by the styloid process and its associated muscles.
2. **What are the main sources of infection for peritonsillar, parapharyngeal, and retropharyngeal abscesses?**
   Peritonsillar abscesses usually arise from an infection of the tonsil or peritonsillar tissue, often as a complication of acute tonsillitis/quinsy. Parapharyngeal abscesses may result from infections in the teeth, tonsils, parotid gland, or pharynx or from penetrating trauma. Retropharyngeal abscesses can occur from infections in the nasopharynx, oropharynx, or paranasal sinuses or from penetrating trauma or instrumentation.
3. **What are the most common organisms causing deep neck infections?**
   Deep neck infections are commonly polymicrobial, involving aerobic and anaerobic bacteria. The most common organisms include *Streptococcus pyogenes*, *Staphylococcus aureus*, *Haemophilus influenzae*, and anaerobes such as *Prevotella*, *Fusobacterium*, and *Bacteroides* species.
4. **What are the potential complications of untreated or inadequately treated deep neck infections?**
   Complications may include airway compromise, sepsis, mediastinitis, carotid artery erosion or thrombosis, jugular vein thrombosis (Lemierre's syndrome: septic thrombophlebitis of the internal jugular vein and metastatic abscesses), necrotizing fasciitis, aspiration pneumonia, empyema, and abscess extension into the neck, thorax, or cranium. Cranial nerve involvement and carotid blowout are rare complications.
5. **How can you differentiate between a peritonsillar abscess and peritonsillar cellulitis?**
   Peritonsillar cellulitis is an inflammation of the peritonsillar tissue without the formation of a discrete abscess. Patients with peritonsillar cellulitis typically present with fever, sore throat, and muffled voice but lack the fluctuance or distinct mass associated with an abscess. Trismus is also much more associated with the abscess formation due to irritation of the pterygoid muscle. Additionally, imaging studies such as CT or ultrasound can help differentiate between cellulitis and an abscess by revealing the presence or absence of a fluid collection.
6. **How is the parapharyngeal space divided?**
   It is divided into two parts by the fascial condensation called the aponeurosis of Zuckerkandl and Testut (stylopharyngeal fascia) joining the *styloid process* to the tensor veli palatini.

7. **What are the contents of parapharyngeal space?**
   - Prestyloid: deep lobe of parotid, medial pterygoid muscle, and mandibular division of trigeminal nerve
   - Poststyloid: IJV; ICA; cranial nerves IX, X, XI, and XII; and sympathetic trunk
8. **What are the layers between the posterior pharyngeal wall vertebrae?**
   From anterior to posterior: buccopharyngeal facia → retropharyngeal space → prevertebral fascia → prevertebral space.
9. **What is the most common route of spread of infection to retropharyngeal space in children?**
   In young children, retropharyngeal abscess may occur due to upper respiratory tract infection spreading to medial retropharyngeal lymph node of Henle. These lymph nodes become rudimentary in the later childhood.
10. **What should you request in your microbiology form?**
    Culture and sensitivity including anaerobic, TB, and atypical mycobacteria (due to the possibility of cold abscess especially in the retropharyngeal abscess)

6.6 Cortical Mastoidectomy

Indications for Surgery [6]

- Chronic or recurrent mastoiditis unresponsive to medical treatment
- Cholesteatoma
- Complications of otitis media (e.g. brain abscess, lateral sinus thrombosis)
- Access for cochlear implantation
- Access to the facial nerve in facial nerve decompression surgery

Specific Risks Involved with the Surgery [6]

- Injury to the facial nerve
- Hearing loss
- Dizziness or vertigo
- Infection
- Bleeding
- Cerebrospinal fluid leak
- Meningitis
- Anaesthesia complications

Steps of the Surgery

1. Preparation: Administer appropriate anaesthesia (usually general anaesthesia), secure the airway, and position the patient supine or lateral decubitus with the affected ear upward.
2. Exposure: Make a postauricular incision, and elevate the skin and periosteum to expose the mastoid bone.
3. Mastoid cortex removal: Use a high-speed drill to remove the mastoid cortex and create a cavity, taking care not to injure the underlying structures such as the sigmoid sinus, dura mater, and facial nerve. The landmark for the mastoid fossa is outlined by MacEwen's triangle (superior: supramastoid crest which is an extension of the posterior root of zygomatic process; anterior: spine of Henle; posterior: hypothetical line tangential to the midpoint of the posterior wall of EAC).
4. Identify and dissect the mastoid air cells, and remove the infected or diseased tissue. If necessary, perform a posterior tympanotomy to access the middle ear and remove any disease or cholesteatoma.
5. Facial nerve identification: Identify the facial nerve using a facial nerve monitor, and protect it throughout the procedure.
6. Wound closure: Irrigate the mastoid cavity with saline, and close the incision using absorbable sutures. Apply a corrugated drain (if subperiosteal abscess) +/− sterile dressing and pressure bandage.
7. Post-operative care: Monitor the patient closely for any signs of complications, such as infection, facial nerve injury, or hearing loss. Manage pain and inflammation with appropriate medications.

Important Points to Note During the Surgery

- Understand the relevant anatomy, including the location of the facial nerve, ossicles, and other structures.
- Be vigilant for potential complications, such as facial nerve injury or worsening infection.
- Preserve as much of the hearing function and facial nerve function as possible to optimize post-operative outcomes.

Questions a Consultant Might Ask a Trainee About the Operation

1. **What is the purpose of a cortical mastoidectomy?**
   The purpose of a cortical mastoidectomy is to remove infected or diseased tissue from the mastoid air cells and create a communication between the mastoid cavity and the middle ear to facilitate drainage and healing.
2. **How can you identify the facial nerve during a cortical mastoidectomy?**
   The facial nerve can be identified by its relationship to the lateral semicircular canal and the mastoid tip. A facial nerve monitor can also be used to help locate and protect the facial nerve during surgery.
3. **How can you minimize the risk of facial nerve injury during a cortical mastoidectomy?**
   To minimize the risk of facial nerve injury, it is essential to understand the relevant anatomy, use a facial nerve monitor, review the CT images thoroughly, and employ careful dissection techniques to avoid damaging the facial nerve.
4. **When would you consider performing a modified radical mastoidectomy instead of a cortical mastoidectomy?**
   A modified radical mastoidectomy would be considered in cases where there is more extensive disease, such as a large cholesteatoma or severe complications from chronic otitis media, that cannot be adequately managed with a cortical mastoidectomy alone, e.g. lateral semicircular canal fistula, extensive tegmen defect, and multiple cholesteatoma recurrences. In a modified radical mastoidectomy, the posterior canal wall and middle ear structures are more extensively removed, and the tympanic membrane is reconstructed.
5. **What type of drill can be used in a cortical mastoidectomy, and what speed setting should be considered?**
   Large cutting burr (5–7 mm): A diamond 1–2 mm burr is considered close to important structures such as the facial nerve. The speed is variable with a maximum speed of 90,000 rev/min. 45,000 rev/min is classically used.
6. **What are the indications of posterior tympanotomy?**
   Cochlear implantation
   Middle ear implants
   Cholesteatoma management as part of a combined approach tympanoplasty
7. **How can you identify the mastoid antrum?**
   About 1.5–3 cm deep to MacEwen's triangle which is bounded by the following: inferiorly: postero-superior margin of EAC, superiorly: temporalis line (suprameatal crest), and posteriorly: a tangential line crossing the EAC and temporalis line (do not confuse with Koerner's septum which is the extension of the petrosquamous suture into the mastoid).
8. **What is the spine of Henle? What is its importance?**
   The spine of Henle is an important landmark found at the posterior superior lateral edge of the ear canal, which marks the level of the antrum of the mastoid. It is present in about 85% of the population.

9. **What is Citelli's angle?**

   The Citelli's angle (sinodural angle) is formed by the tegmen superiorly and the transverse sinus inferiorly. Sigmoid sinus is the continuation of the transverse sinus at this point. Drilling of that angle exposes the bony landmarks of the cortical mastoidectomy (dural plate and sigmoid plate) and improves access to deeper structures.

6.7 Evacuation of an Orbital Subperiosteal Abscess (Complication of Acute Sinusitis)

Indications for Surgery

- Persistent or worsening symptoms despite appropriate medical management.
- Signs of orbital or intracranial complications (e.g. proptosis, vision loss, cranial nerve deficits).
- Large or loculated subperiosteal abscess visible on imaging. See Fig. 6.8.

Specific Risks Involved with the Surgery

- Bleeding
- Infection
- Injury to adjacent structures (e.g. orbital contents, sinuses)
- Recurrence of the abscess
- Anaesthesia complications

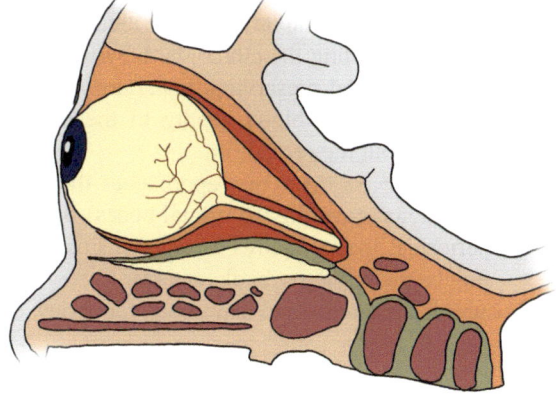

Fig. 6.8 Subperiosteal abscess formation. Illustrated by Vikum Liyanaarachchi

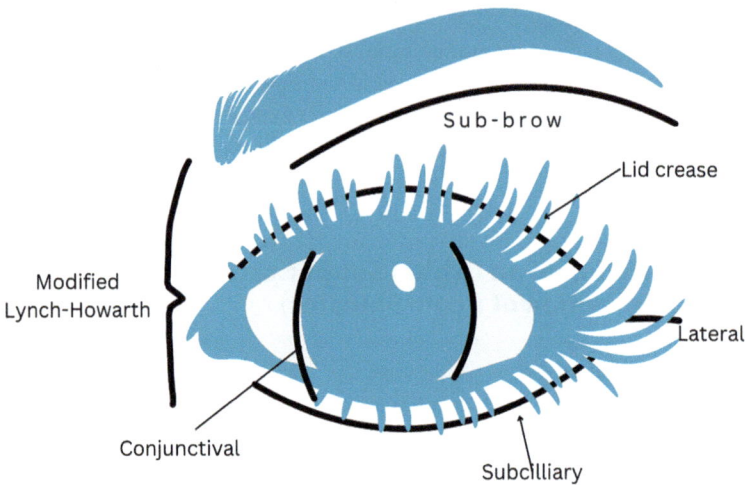

Fig. 6.9 Different incisions which can be performed to access orbital abscess. Illustrated by Vikum Liyanaarachchi

Steps of the Surgery

External Approach: Lynch-Howarth Incision (Fig. 6.9)
1. Preparation: Administer appropriate anaesthesia (usually general anaesthesia), and position the patient supine with the head elevated.
2. Incision: The Lynch-Howarth incision is made along the medial aspect of the upper eyelid, following the curvature of the bony orbit. It may extend from the area near the bridge of the nose across the eyebrow, allowing access to the ethmoidal sinuses and the orbit's medial wall.
3. Dissection: The dissection proceeds through the skin and subcutaneous tissues, followed by the careful separation of the orbicularis oculi muscle to expose the periosteum of the orbital rim. Careful subperiosteal dissection allows access to the subperiosteal space without entering the orbital cavity itself.
    Structures encountered:
    (a) Anterior ethmoidal artery: A critical landmark, the anterior ethmoidal artery runs along the ethmoidal labyrinth and is at risk during dissection. Identifying and preserving this artery are crucial to prevent bleeding and ensure adequate blood supply to the orbital structures. Typically seen 24 mm from the orbital rim.
    (b) Periorbita: As dissection approaches the orbital wall, the periorbita (the periosteum covering the orbital bones) is encountered. Entry into the subperiosteal space requires careful incision of the periorbita without damaging the underlying orbital contents.
4. Closure: Place a drain and leave open for review the following day.

Endoscopic Approach: Sinus Surgery

1. Access to the subperiosteal abscess is gained endoscopically through the nasal cavity, utilizing natural nasal passages and sinus openings. This approach often involves functional endoscopic sinus surgery (FESS) to address any underlying sinusitis contributing to the abscess formation.
2. Landmarks for lamina papyracea:
   - The procedure begins with endoscopic visualization of the nasal cavity, identifying key anatomical landmarks such as the middle turbinate, uncinate process, and ethmoid bulla.
3. Accessing the ethmoid sinus:
   - A careful uncinectomy and anterior ethmoidectomy are performed to expose the ethmoid sinus air cells and to approach the lamina papyracea safely.
   - The lamina papyracea serves as the lateral boundary of the ethmoid sinuses and the medial wall of the orbit, making it a critical landmark in this procedure.
4. Identification and management of the lamina papyracea:
   - The lamina papyracea is identified as a thin, delicate bone separating the ethmoid air cells from the orbital contents. Surgeons must exercise caution to preserve its integrity while accessing the subperiosteal space.
   - In cases where the abscess is pressing against the lamina papyracea, slight bulging may be noted. The approach to the lamina papyracea may involve gentle manipulation or careful removal of a small portion to create an access point to the abscess.
5. Evacuating the abscess:
   - Once access through the lamina papyracea is secured, this can be done by using a curette or ball seeker probe, and the subperiosteal abscess can be approached.
   - The objective is to achieve complete drainage of the abscess while avoiding any injury to the orbital contents, including the optic nerve and extraocular muscles.
6. Ensuring adequate drainage:
   - Following abscess evacuation, the surgeon may ensure that adequate drainage is established to prevent recurrence. This could involve creating a small fenestration in the lamina papyracea that allows continued drainage of any residual infection into the nasal cavity.
7. Post-operative care: Administer appropriate antibiotics, analgesics, and anti-inflammatory medications. Monitor the patient closely for any signs of complications, such as infection, bleeding, or recurrence of the abscess.

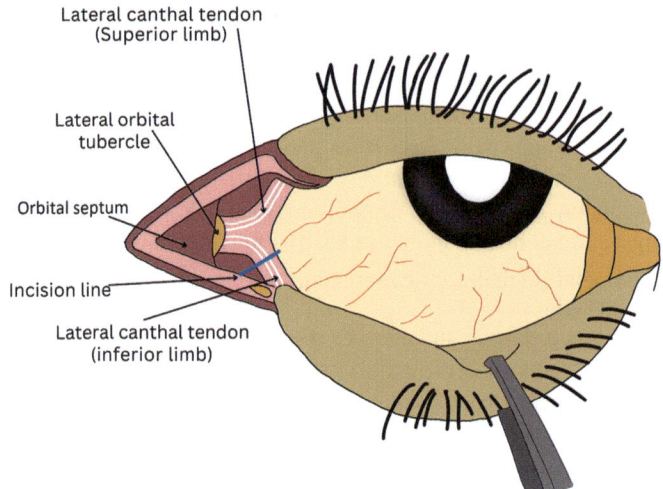

Fig. 6.10 Lateral canthotomy anatomy and incision of inferior limb marked. Illustrated by Vikum Liyanaarachchi

Important Points to Note During the Surgery

- Carefully assess the location and extent of the abscess using preoperative imaging to guide the surgical approach.
- Take care to avoid injury to adjacent structures, such as the orbital contents or sinuses.
- Ensure adequate drainage and ventilation of the affected sinuses to reduce the risk of recurrence.
- Consider lateral cantholysis/canthotomy to reduce eye pressure (Fig. 6.10).

Questions a Consultant Might Ask a Trainee About the Operation

1. **What are the main complications of acute sinusitis that may necessitate surgical intervention?**
   The main complications include subperiosteal abscess, orbital cellulitis, and intracranial complications, such as meningitis or abscess formation.
2. **What factors should be considered when selecting a surgical approach for evacuating a subperiosteal abscess?**
   Factors to consider include the location and size of the abscess, the presence of concurrent sinusitis, and the surgeon's familiarity and experience with the selected approach. Also the patient's input is important.
3. **What are some potential complications of evacuating a subperiosteal abscess?**
   Potential complications include bleeding, infection, injury to adjacent structures (e.g. orbital contents, sinuses), recurrence of the abscess, and anaesthesia complications.

4. When should a surgeon consider performing sinus surgery in conjunction with evacuating a subperiosteal abscess?

   A surgeon should consider performing sinus surgery in conjunction with evacuating a subperiosteal abscess if the abscess is secondary to acute sinusitis and if medical management has failed to resolve the underlying sinusitis.

5. **Is there any role for conservative medical management of subperiosteal abscess?**

   There is evidence that small abscess 3–4 mm or less and proptosis 5 mm or less with no significant ocular signs could be treated conservatively with similar outcome to surgery.

6. **What is Chandler classification?**
   - Stage 1: Preseptal cellulitis
   - Stage 2: Orbital cellulitis
   - Stage 3: Subperiosteal abscess
   - Stage 4: Orbital abscess
   - Stage 5: Cavernous sinus thrombosis

7. **When do you consider requesting urgent imaging in children with orbital complications of sinusitis?**
   - Suspecting post-septal disease (Chandler's II–V)
   - Marked reduced eye opening
   - Reduced eye movements
   - Marked chemosis, proptosis, ophthalmoplegia
   - Any neurological signs
   - No improvement in general condition or orbital signs or swinging pyrexia after 24–36 h of appropriate medical treatment

8. **In an external approach, what are the important landmarks to consider?**

   The key structures found with this approach are summarized with the rule of halves from the orbital rim/lacrimal sac: the anterior ethmoid artery is found 24 mm posterior to the anterior lacrimal crest, then the posterior ethmoid artery is another 12 mm, and the optic nerve is found a further 6 mm.

9. **What is the orbital septum?**
   - It is a fibrous membrane that lies deep to the orbicularis oculi muscle extending from the periosteum of the orbit to the levator aponeurosis in the upper eyelid and to the inferior border of the tarsal plate in the lower eyelid.
   - It acts as a barrier to the spread of infection from skin and subcutaneous tissues into the orbit.

6.8 Arrest of Post-Tonsillar Haemorrhage

Indications for Surgery

- Primary or secondary post-tonsillectomy bleeding
- Uncontrolled bleeding from the tonsillar bed or area
- Haemodynamic instability or significant blood loss due to tonsillar bleeding

Specific Risks Involved with the Surgery

- Bleeding
- Infection
- Injury to adjacent structures (e.g. nerves, blood vessels)
- Aspiration of blood or secretions
- Anaesthesia complications

Steps of the Surgery

1. Preparation: Administer appropriate anaesthesia (usually general anaesthesia), and position the patient supine with the head elevated and the neck extended.
2. Visualization and control of the bleeding site: (a) Suction any blood or secretions from the oral cavity to visualize the bleeding site. (b) Apply direct pressure with a moistened gauze or sponge to the bleeding site to achieve initial haemostasis.
3. Haemostasis: (a) Identify the bleeding vessel or source of haemorrhage. (b) Perform haemostasis using electrocautery, suture ligation, or surgical clips, as appropriate for the bleeding source. If the bleeding cannot be stopped using cautery, then using a straight Birkett's forceps, grab the bleeding tissue, and then place a Negus forceps behind it; then using a silk tie, you can ligate the bleeding. If this fails, you can place a haemostatic material in between the tonsil pillars and tie them together. If this also fails, then pack the oropharynx tightly, leave the patient intubated, and consider performing an external carotid artery embolization with the interventional radiology team.
4. Inspection and irrigation: (a) Inspect the tonsillar bed and surrounding area to ensure complete haemostasis and to identify any additional bleeding sources. (b) Irrigate the surgical field with saline to remove any blood clots or debris.
5. Gastric emptying.
6. Post-operative care: Monitor the patient closely for any signs of complications, such as recurrent bleeding, infection, or respiratory distress. Administer appropriate analgesics, anti-inflammatory medications, and antibiotics if indicated.

Important Points to Note During the Surgery

- Quickly and effectively secure the airway to minimize the risk of aspiration.
- Take care to identify and preserve vital structures, such as nerves and blood vessels, during the procedure.
- Ensure complete haemostasis before concluding the surgery to prevent recurrent bleeding.

Questions a Consultant Might Ask a Trainee About the Operation

1. **What are the main causes of acute tonsillar haemorrhage?**
   The main causes of acute tonsillar haemorrhage include primary or secondary post-tonsillectomy bleeding, trauma, and spontaneous bleeding from an underlying vascular anomaly or coagulopathy.
2. **What factors can increase the risk of post-tonsillectomy bleeding?**
   Factors that can increase the risk of post-tonsillectomy bleeding include inadequate intraoperative haemostasis, infection, patient non-compliance with post-operative instructions, and underlying coagulopathy.
3. **How can you differentiate primary from secondary post-tonsillectomy bleeding?**
   Primary post-tonsillectomy bleeding occurs within the first 24 h after surgery and is typically due to inadequate intraoperative haemostasis, while secondary post-tonsillectomy bleeding occurs more than 24 h after surgery and is often related to infection, inflammation, or sloughing of the eschar.
4. **What are the potential complications of surgical management of acute tonsillar haemorrhage?**
   Potential complications include bleeding, infection, injury to adjacent structures (e.g. nerves, blood vessels), aspiration of blood or secretions, and anaesthesia complications.
5. **What measures can be taken to prevent post-tonsillectomy bleeding?**
   Measures to prevent post-tonsillectomy bleeding include careful intraoperative haemostasis, appropriate post-operative pain control, patient education on post-operative instructions, and identification and management of any underlying coagulopathy.
6. **What is the blood supply of the palatine tonsil?**
   Arterial: All from external carotid artery system.
   - Dorsal lingual artery from the lingual artery
   - Ascending palatine artery from the facial artery
   - Tonsillar branch of the facial artery
   - Ascending pharyngeal artery of the external carotid artery
   - Lesser palatine artery of the descending palatine artery, a branch of the maxillary artery
   Venous:
   - Peritonsillar plexus of veins. This plexus drains into the pharyngeal and lingual veins, which drain into the internal jugular vein.
7. **Why gastric emptying is important in post-tonsillectomy bleeding?**
   To avoid Mendelson's syndrome which is characterized by a bronchopulmonary reaction following aspiration of gastric contents during general anaesthesia due to abolition of the laryngeal reflexes. It may end up with pulmonary oedema.

8. **What anaesthetic technique is used during induction of anaesthesia in patients with post-tonsillectomy bleeding?**

    Rapid sequence induction and intubation are a technique designed to minimize the chance of pulmonary aspiration. This involves cricoid pressure (Sellick manoeuvre) during induction and intubation.

9. **If external carotid artery ligation is warranted, what are the anatomical landmarks?**

    External carotid artery (ECA) is the branching artery. Identify at least two branches to make sure that it is the external carotid. One can ligate the branches or the main trunk of ECA. ECA lies medial, while internal carotid is lateral. The origin of the ECA can be marked by joining two points: the first on the anterior edge of the sternocleidomastoid muscle at the upper level of the thyroid cartilage and the second point on the posterior border of the neck of the mandible.

6.9 Surgical Management of Ludwig's Angina

Indications for Surgery

- Rapidly progressing infection with airway compromise
- Inadequate response to conservative management (e.g. antibiotics, drainage)
- Development of complications, such as abscess formation or mediastinitis

Specific Risks Involved with the Surgery

- Bleeding
- Infection
- Injury to adjacent structures (e.g. nerves, blood vessels, salivary ducts)
- Aspiration of secretions or pus
- Anaesthesia complications

Steps of the Surgery

1. Preparation: Administer appropriate anaesthesia (usually general anaesthesia), and secure the airway with endotracheal intubation or a surgical airway if necessary. Position the patient supine with the head elevated and the neck extended.
2. Incision and exposure:
    (a) Make a horizontal incision or multiple free incisions in the submandibular region, just below the lower border of the mandible (Fig. 6.11).
    (b) Dissect through the subcutaneous tissue and platysma muscle, taking care to preserve the marginal mandibular branch of the facial nerve.
3. Drainage of the infection:
    (a) Locate the involved submandibular and sublingual spaces by careful blunt dissection (see Fig. 6.12).

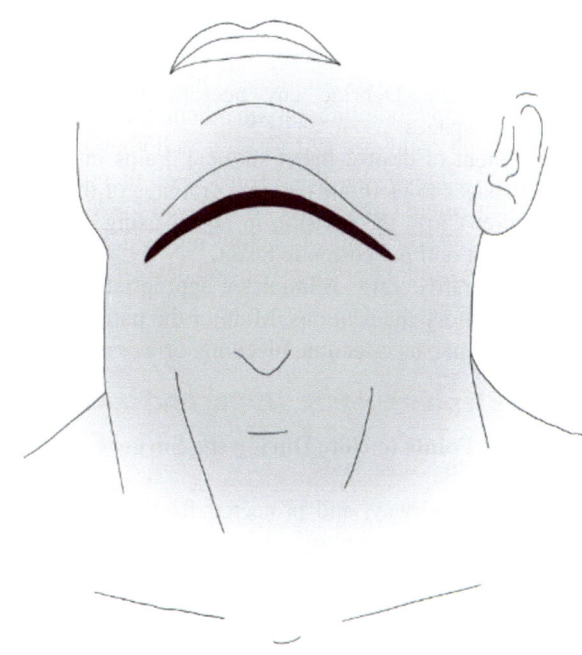

Fig. 6.11 Ludwig's angina classical incision. Illustrated by Vikum Liyanaarachchi

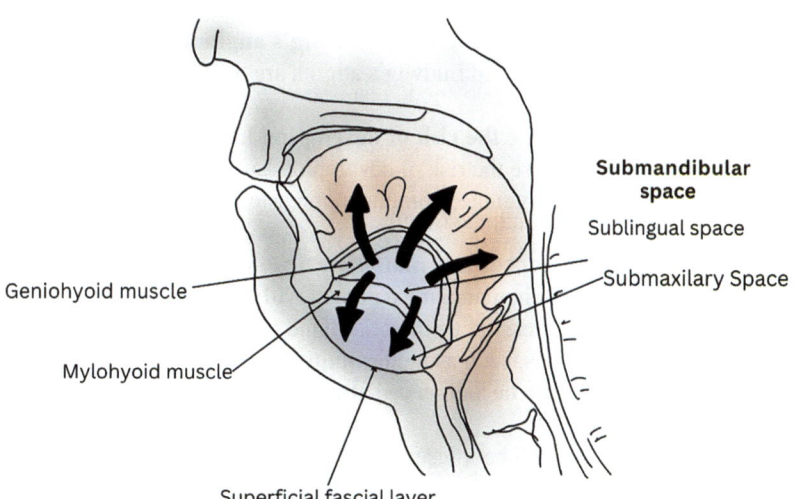

Fig. 6.12 Anatomy of Ludwig's angina showing abscess formation. Illustrated by Vikum Liyanaarachchi

(b) Incise the fascial layers covering the involved spaces to drain the infection.
   (c) Break down any loculations within the spaces using a finger or blunt instrument.
4. Debridement: Debride any necrotic tissue or foreign material from the infected spaces.
5. Placement of drains: Insert surgical drains into the submandibular and sublingual spaces to facilitate ongoing drainage of the infection.
6. Closure: Close the incision in layers using absorbable sutures, taking care to obtain an optimal cosmetic result.
7. Post-operative care: Administer appropriate antibiotics, analgesics, and anti-inflammatory medications. Monitor the patient closely for any signs of complications, such as infection, bleeding, or worsening airway compromise.

Important Points to Note During the Surgery

- Secure the airway, and protect it from aspiration of secretions or pus—may require a tracheostomy or the patient may need to remain intubated post-operatively.
- Take care to preserve vital structures, such as nerves, blood vessels, and salivary ducts.
- Ensure adequate drainage of the involved spaces to prevent recurrence of the infection.

Questions a Consultant Might Ask a Trainee About the Operation

1. **What are the main spaces involved in Ludwig's angina?**
   The main spaces involved in Ludwig's angina are the bilateral submandibular and sublingual spaces.
2. **What factors can increase the risk of developing Ludwig's angina?**
   Factors that can increase the risk of developing Ludwig's angina include dental infections, poor oral hygiene, immunosuppression, and underlying systemic diseases (e.g. diabetes).
3. **What are the primary concerns in managing a patient with Ludwig's angina?**
   The primary concerns in managing a patient with Ludwig's angina are airway compromise, rapid progression of infection, and potential development of life-threatening complications, such as mediastinitis or sepsis.
4. **What structures should be preserved during the surgical management of Ludwig's angina?**
   Structures that should be preserved during the surgical management of Ludwig's angina include the marginal mandibular branch of the facial nerve, blood vessels, and salivary ducts.

5. **What is the role of surgical management in the treatment of Ludwig's angina?**
   The role of surgical management in the treatment of Ludwig's angina is to rapidly drain the infection, relieve pressure on the airway, and prevent the development of life-threatening complications, such as mediastinitis or sepsis.
6. **What are the most common organisms involved in Ludwig's angina?**
   It is usually multiple organisms including Gram positive, Gram negative, and anaerobes. The most common organisms involved include *Streptococcus viridans* and *Staphylococcus aureus*.
7. **How can Ludwig's angina cause airway compromise?**
   Extension of infection in the sublingual space above the mylohyoid muscle, and submandibular space below the mylohyoid muscle. This will lead to elevation of the tongue and obstruct the airway. In addition, associated upper airway oedema and lymphadenoma may contribute to the airway compromise. Airway compromise can occur within 1–2 h of initial presentation.

6.10 Emergency Endoscopic Sinus Surgery (for Complications of Acute Sinusitis, Such as Orbital or Intracranial Abscess)

Indications for Surgery

- Complications of acute sinusitis, such as orbital cellulitis, subperiosteal abscess, orbital abscess, or intracranial abscess
- Inadequate response to conservative management (e.g. antibiotics, drainage)
- Significant sinonasal polyposis or anatomic abnormalities contributing to the sinusitis

Specific Risks Involved with the Surgery

- Bleeding
- Infection
- Injury to adjacent structures (e.g. orbital contents, skull base, sinuses)
- Recurrence of the infection
- Anaesthesia complications

Steps of the Surgery

1. Preparation:
   (a) Administer general anaesthesia, and position the patient supine with the head elevated, optimizing access to the nasal cavity.
   (b) Apply topical vasoconstrictors and decongestants to the nasal mucosa to minimize bleeding and improve visibility.

2. Endoscopic access and visualization:
   (a) Insert a rigid endoscope into the nasal cavity, advancing it through the middle meatus for optimal visualization, and medialize the middle turbinate.
   (b) Clear any obstructions in the nasal cavity using suction devices or forceps, such as polyps, mucus, or debris.
   (c) Identify key anatomical landmarks including the uncinate process, ethmoid bulla, and middle turbinate.
   (d) Access the ethmoid sinuses, carefully handling the lamina papyracea. Thinning out or cautiously opening the lamina papyracea is essential if it is intact, ensuring not to damage the periorbita or orbital contents.
3. Opening the affected sinuses:
   (a) Identify the ostia of the affected sinuses. Enlarge the openings using sinus curettes or powered instrumentation for adequate drainage and ventilation.
4. Drainage of orbital abscess:
   (a) If an orbital abscess is present, decompression of the orbit by carefully removing part of the lamina papyracea (as mentioned in the previous section) can be performed; this will also help with drainage of the abscess.
   (b) Drain the abscess by incising the abscess wall and evacuating the pus using suction or curettes.

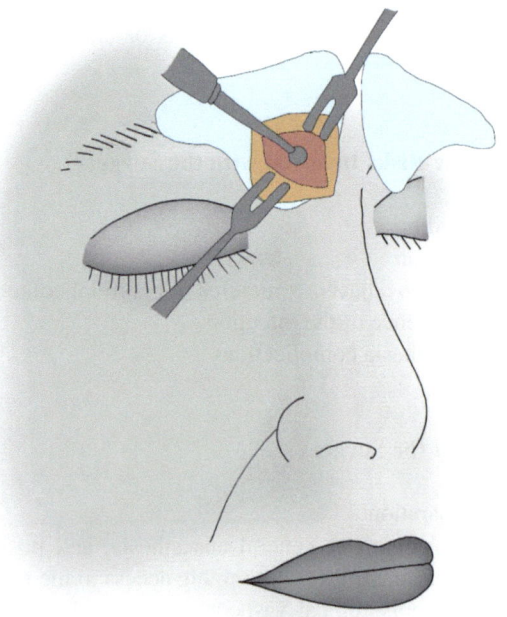

Fig. 6.13 Surgical drill being used to enter the frontal sinus. Illustrated by Vikum Liyanaarachchi

Drainage of Intracranial Abscess Secondary to Frontal Sinus

1. Marking and Incision:
   - A small, precise incision is marked on the skin directly over the frontal sinus, typically about 1 cm above the eyebrow. Care is taken to ensure that the location corresponds accurately to the underlying frontal sinus, using palpation or preoperative imaging for guidance.
   - The incision is made through the skin and subcutaneous tissue to expose the periosteum.
2. Creating the Burr Hole (Trephination):
   - The periosteum is incised and elevated to expose the outer table of the frontal bone.
   - A surgical drill or trephine is used to create a burr hole through the outer table of the frontal sinus (Fig. 6.13). This step requires precise control to penetrate the bone without injuring the sinus mucosa or entering the cranial cavity inadvertently.
   - The diameter of the burr hole is typically small, just large enough to facilitate adequate drainage and, if necessary, the introduction of an endoscope for direct visualization.
3. Accessing the Frontal Sinus and Drainage:
   - Once the outer table is breached, the surgeon carefully enters the frontal sinus, taking care to preserve the sinus mucosa as much as possible.
   - Any pus or infectious material within the frontal sinus is gently suctioned out. Samples may be taken for microbiological analysis.
   - If an intracranial extension of the abscess is present and accessible through this approach, further careful dissection and drainage are performed in collaboration with neurosurgery.
4. Ensuring Adequate Drainage:
   - The surgeon may choose to insert a small tube or stent into the trephine opening to maintain sinus drainage post-operatively. This ensures continued ventilation and drainage of the frontal sinus, reducing the risk of re-accumulation of pus.
5. Closure:
   - A drainage tube is placed; it is secured and dressed appropriately.

Post-operative Care

- Administer appropriate antibiotics, analgesics, and anti-inflammatory medications.
- Monitor the patient closely for signs of complications, such as infection, bleeding, or worsening of the condition.

Important Points to Note During the Surgery

- Take care to avoid injury to adjacent structures, such as the orbital contents or skull base.
- Ensure adequate drainage and ventilation of the affected sinuses to reduce the risk of recurrence.
- In the case of an orbital or intracranial abscess, ensure appropriate drainage and avoid complications.

Questions a Consultant Might Ask a Trainee About the Operation

1. **What are some common complications of acute sinusitis that may necessitate emergency endoscopic sinus surgery?**
   Complications of acute sinusitis that may necessitate emergency endoscopic sinus surgery include orbital cellulitis, subperiosteal abscess, orbital abscess, or intracranial abscess.
2. **In cases of orbital abscess or intracranial complications due to acute sinusitis, what are the indications for emergency endoscopic sinus surgery?**
   Indications for emergency endoscopic sinus surgery in cases of orbital abscess or intracranial complications due to acute sinusitis include failure of medical treatment (e.g. antibiotics and/or corticosteroids), significant visual disturbances, progression of infection or abscess, and/or presence of neurological symptoms or signs of intracranial extension.
3. **What are some important anatomic landmarks within the sinuses that a surgeon should be familiar with during emergency endoscopic sinus surgery?**
   Important anatomic landmarks within the sinuses include the middle turbinate, uncinate process, ethmoid bulla, osteomeatal complex, and anterior skull base.
4. **How can you minimize the risk of complications during emergency endoscopic sinus surgery?**
   To minimize the risk of complications during emergency endoscopic sinus surgery, ensure adequate visualization, maintain a good understanding of the sinus anatomy, avoid injury to adjacent structures, and ensure adequate drainage and ventilation of the affected sinuses.
5. **What is the role of post-operative care in the management of patients undergoing emergency endoscopic sinus surgery?**
   Post-operative care in the management of patients undergoing emergency endoscopic sinus surgery includes administering appropriate antibiotics, analgesics, and anti-inflammatory medications; monitoring for complications; and ensuring proper follow-up care to evaluate sinus function and healing.
6. **Do you know any categorization of the ethmoidal roof?**
   Keros classification:
   - **Type 1**: olfactory fossa 1–3 mm deep
   - **Type 2**: olfactory fossa 4–7 mm deep

- **Type 3**: olfactory fossa 8–16 mm
- **Type 4** (not in the original classification but used to describe **olfactory fossa with asymmetric skull base**)

7. **What are important landmarks seen on CT for endoscopic sinus surgery?**
   - C—Cribriform plate
   - L—Lamina (lamina papyracea and lateral lamella: Keros)
   - O—Optic nerve/Onodi cells
   - S—Sphenoid (sellar, presellar, postsellar 70–75%, conchal 0–5%)
   - E—Ethmoid artery (Kennedy's nipple)
   - D—Dentition/teeth

(Refer to FESS questions in Rhinology, Chap. 3)

6.11 Surgical Decompression of Facial Nerve

Indications for Surgery

- Acute facial paralysis due to severe infection (e.g. Bell's palsy with poor recovery, Ramsay Hunt syndrome)
- Facial paralysis secondary to trauma (e.g. temporal bone fracture, penetrating injury, or iatrogenic)
- Facial paralysis caused by a neoplasm (e.g. schwannoma, parotid gland tumour)

Risks Involved with the Surgery

- Infection
- Bleeding
- Persistent or worsened facial paralysis
- Hearing loss
- Taste disturbance

Steps of the Surgery

1. Facial nerve function evaluation: Conduct a detailed assessment of the patient's facial nerve function to document any preoperative deficits.
2. Cause of paralysis identification: Utilize high-resolution CT scans of the temporal bone to localize the fracture and assess its impact on the facial nerve. MRI may be employed to evaluate soft tissue and nerve integrity.
3. General anaesthesia is administered to ensure patient comfort and immobility throughout the procedure.
4. Positioning: The patient is positioned supine with the head turned away from the operative side, slightly extended to enhance temporal bone access.

5. Incision and exposure:
   - Postauricular mastoidectomy incision: A postauricular incision is made, like that for a mastoidectomy, extending from the mastoid tip to above the ear level for sufficient surgical field exposure.
6. Facial nerve and landmark identification:
   - Key landmarks such as the mastoid antrum, sigmoid sinus, and digastric ridge are identified. The facial nerve is carefully traced from the stylomastoid foramen, monitoring its course relative to the temporal bone fracture.
7. Decompression:
   - Evaluating and addressing the fracture: The extent of the fracture's involvement with the fallopian canal, housing the facial nerve, is assessed. Compressive elements like bone fragments are meticulously removed.
8. Bony fallopian canal skeletonization: The facial nerve is decompressed by delicately skeletonizing the bony canal to relieve any pressure, avoiding direct nerve manipulation to prevent additional trauma. Carefully perform with a curette or diamond burr drill.
9. Closure
   - Layered wound closure: After achieving haemostasis, the surgical site is closed in layers—starting with the periosteum, followed by the soft tissue, and finally the skin, employing fine suturing techniques for optimal healing and aesthetic results.
10. Post-operative care:
    - Facial nerve function monitoring: Regular post-operative evaluations of facial nerve function are essential to assess recovery and identify any potential deterioration.
    - Complication management: Vigilance for infection, haematoma, or cerebrospinal fluid leak is maintained, with prompt management of any issues encountered.
    - Rehabilitation: Patients are encouraged to participate in facial rehabilitation exercises and, if necessary, referred for further specialist evaluation and treatment to support recovery.

Important Points to Note During the Surgery

- Meticulous dissection and identification of the facial nerve and its branches are crucial to minimize the risk of injury.
- Intraoperative nerve monitoring may be used to help identify and protect the facial nerve during dissection.
- Adequate haemostasis is essential to prevent post-operative haematoma and facilitate wound healing.
- If the cause of paralysis is a neoplasm, ensure complete removal of the tumour while preserving as much facial nerve function as possible.

6 Emergencies

Questions a Consultant Might Ask a Trainee About the Operation

1. **What imaging studies can be helpful in evaluating a patient with facial paralysis before surgery?**
   MRI and CT scans can help identify the cause of facial paralysis (e.g. trauma, tumour, infection) and assess the extent of nerve compression or damage.
2. **How can intraoperative nerve monitoring be useful during surgical decompression of the facial nerve?**
   Intraoperative nerve monitoring can help identify and protect the facial nerve during dissection, reducing the risk of iatrogenic injury and improving surgical outcomes.
3. **How many segments are there of the facial nerve at the mastoid bone? What are they called?**
   Within the mastoid bone, the facial nerve traverses through several anatomically distinct segments after exiting the brainstem and before reaching its peripheral branches. There are four well-defined segments:
   (a) Meatal segment (internal auditory canal—IAC):
       Length: Approximately 8–10 mm
       This segment lies within the IAC alongside the vestibulocochlear nerve (CN VIII). It begins at the brainstem and ends at the fundus of the IAC, just before entering the labyrinthine segment.
   (b) Labyrinthine segment:
       Length: Approximately 3–5 mm
       It is the shortest and narrowest portion of the facial nerve, running from the fundus of the IAC to the geniculate ganglion. This segment makes a sharp turn (first genu) at the geniculate ganglion. It is highly susceptible to ischemic injuries due to its narrow bony canal and vascular supply.
   (c) Tympanic segment (horizontal segment):
       Length: Approximately 11 mm
       This extends from the geniculate ganglion to the second sharp bend (second genu). It runs horizontally across the medial wall of the middle ear, above the oval window, making it susceptible to middle ear pathologies.
   (d) Mastoid segment (vertical segment):
       Length: Approximately 13 mm
       It runs vertically downward from the second genu to the stylomastoid foramen. This segment traverses the mastoid bone and is the segment most frequently exposed during mastoidectomy procedures. It is the area where the nerve is most vulnerable to iatrogenic injury during ear surgeries.
   Clinical Relevance
   - Bell's palsy and the geniculate ganglion: In Bell's palsy, a common form of facial nerve paralysis, the geniculate ganglion (just after the first genu) is often implicated as the site of nerve inflammation and compression within its narrow bony canal. This segment's susceptibility is attributed to the anatomical constraints and vascular supply that may predispose it to ischaemic injury.

- Iatrogenic injuries and the second genu: Surgical procedures involving the mastoid bone or middle ear, such as mastoidectomy, pose a risk to the facial nerve, particularly at the second genu where the nerve makes a sharp turn from the tympanic segment to the mastoid segment. This area is at risk due to its proximity to surgical fields in common otologic procedures.

4. **What is the clinical classification for facial nerve palsy?**

    House-Brackmann classification from I to VI is one of the commonest used classifications in which I is normal and VI is complete disfigurement. In I, II, and III, there is complete eye closure, while IV, V, and VI showed incomplete closure of the eyelid. It depends on static and dynamic assessment of the different branches of the facial nerve. Sunnybrook and Sydney are two other classifications also used.

5. **How can you clinically determine the level of a facial nerve injury?**

    Determining the level of facial nerve injury clinically involves a series of tests that can help pinpoint the site of lesion along the nerve's anatomical course. These tests are designed to assess the function of specific branches of the facial nerve, thereby providing clues to the location of the injury.

    (a) Schirmer Test

    This test measures tear production to assess the function of the lacrimal gland, which is innervated by the greater superficial petrosal nerve, a branch of the facial nerve.

    A decrease in tear production (indicative of defective lacrimation) on the affected side suggests an injury proximal to the geniculate ganglion, where the greater superficial petrosal nerve branches off from the main trunk of the facial nerve.

    This test is specifically useful for identifying lesions affecting the facial nerve before it branches at the geniculate ganglion.

    (b) Stapedial Reflex Assessment with Tympanometry

    This evaluates the acoustic reflex, which involves the stapedius muscle in the middle ear. The muscle is innervated by a branch of the facial nerve that arises just proximal to the nerve's second bend (second genu).

    Loss of the stapedial reflex on tympanometry indicates an injury proximal to the second genu of the facial nerve, implicating the segment of the nerve to the stapedius muscle.

    It is useful for diagnosing injuries between the geniculate ganglion and the second bend of the facial nerve, where the branch to the stapedius muscle originates.

    (c) Gustatory Flow Rate Measurement

    This assesses salivation as a measure of chorda tympani nerve function, which carries taste from the anterior two-thirds of the tongue and parasympathetic fibres to the submandibular and sublingual glands.

    A significant reduction in salivation on one side compared to the other may indicate an injury affecting the facial nerve prior to the exit of the chorda tympani (which branches off the facial nerve before it exits the stylomastoid foramen).

This test is particularly indicative of lesions affecting the facial nerve before it branches to the chorda tympani but after the geniculate ganglion.

Additional Considerations

- House-Brackmann scale: While not a specific test for locating the site of injury, this grading system is widely used to assess the severity of facial nerve dysfunction and can complement the above tests in evaluating and managing facial nerve injuries.
- Electrophysiological tests: Electroneuronography (ENoG) and electromyography (EMG) can provide additional quantitative data on the degree and location of nerve injury, especially in acute settings.

6. **What surgical approach could be used for facial nerve exploration?**

    If no serviceable hearing is present: trans-labyrinthine approach: This method is preferred for patients without serviceable hearing. It provides direct access to the internal auditory canal and facial nerve, allowing for thorough exploration and management of facial nerve pathology without the concern of preserving hearing.

    If serviceable hearing is present: The decision-making process involves topographic testing to determine the extent of nerve involvement and guide the choice of surgical approach.

    Topographic Testing Results:

- No lacrimation (positive Schirmer test indicating greater superficial petrosal nerve involvement):
- Middle cranial fossa approach: This approach is indicated when there is evidence of involvement of the facial nerve's branch, the greater superficial petrosal nerve, suggesting pathology that might be accessible through the middle cranial fossa. This method aims to preserve hearing while allowing access to the facial nerve within the temporal bone.

    Preserved lacrimation (negative Schirmer test):

- Transmastoid approach: Preferred when lacrimation is intact, suggesting that the distal segments of the facial nerve are affected. This approach allows for exploration and decompression of the facial nerve via the mastoid, with a focus on preserving both facial function and hearing.

7. **How do different types of fractures affect the ear?**

    A longitudinal fracture (usually from lateral blow, temporal or parietal) typically runs parallel to the external auditory canal, through the middle ear (causing a perforation or haemotympanum), anterior to the otic capsule, and parallel to the petrous ridge, and extending to the foramen ovale. It usually causes conductive hearing loss.

    Transverse fractures run perpendicular to the petrous ridge, from the foramen magnum across the petrous pyramid, often including the internal auditory canal, and into the foramen spinosum or lacerum and usually cause sensorineural hearing loss.

6.12 Drainage of Acute Parotitis or Parotid Abscess

Indications for Surgery

- Acute bacterial parotitis not responding to conservative management (e.g. intravenous antibiotics, hydration, and analgesics).
- Parotid abscess formation.
- High risk of complications, such as facial nerve injury, systemic infection, or sepsis.

Specific Risks Involved with the Surgery

- Infection
- Bleeding
- Injury to the facial nerve
- Injury to surrounding structures (e.g. salivary ducts, blood vessels)
- Recurrence of parotitis or abscess

Steps of the Surgery

- Preoperative assessment: Evaluate the patient's clinical condition, confirm the diagnosis of parotitis or abscess with imaging studies (e.g. ultrasound, CT scan), and administer intravenous antibiotics.
- Anaesthesia: Administer local anaesthesia with or without sedation, or general anaesthesia depending on the patient's condition and preference.
- Positioning: Place the patient in a supine position with the head turned away from the affected side.
- Incision: Perform a modified Blair incision—a curved incision that starts in the preauricular region, extends around the earlobe, and then curves posteriorly into the neck.
- Dissection: Raise subplatysmal flaps to expose the parotid gland.
- Drainage: Identify the abscess or inflamed area, incise the capsule of the parotid gland, and drain the purulent material. Use caution to avoid injuring the facial nerve.
- Irrigation: Irrigate the abscess cavity with sterile saline solution.
- Placement of a drain: Insert a Penrose or closed suction drain into the cavity to prevent fluid accumulation and promote healing.
- Closure: Close the wound in layers with appropriate suturing techniques.
- Post-operative care: Continue intravenous antibiotics, monitor the patient for complications, and remove the drain when output decreases.

Important Points to Note During the Surgery

- Preserve the facial nerve by using meticulous dissection techniques and identifying its branches.
- Use imaging studies, such as ultrasound or CT scan, to help identify the location of the abscess or inflamed area before surgery.
- Ensure adequate drainage and irrigation of the abscess cavity to minimize the risk of recurrent infection.

Questions a Consultant Might Ask a Trainee About the Operation

1. **What is the role of conservative management in acute parotitis or parotid abscess?**
   Conservative management, including intravenous antibiotics, hydration, and analgesics, is the first-line treatment for acute parotitis. Surgical drainage is indicated when conservative measures fail, or there is a risk of complications.
2. **How can imaging studies help in the preoperative assessment of a patient with acute parotitis or parotid abscess?**
   Imaging studies, such as ultrasound or CT scan, can confirm the diagnosis, identify the location and extent of the abscess, and help plan the surgical approach.
3. **What precautions should be taken during the dissection to avoid injury to the facial nerve?**
   Meticulous dissection techniques and knowledge of the facial nerve anatomy are essential. Surgeons should identify and preserve the main trunk and branches of the facial nerve during the procedure.
4. **Why is the placement of a drain important after drainage of a parotid abscess?**
   Placing a drain after drainage of a parotid abscess helps prevent fluid accumulation, promotes healing, and reduces the risk of recurrent infection.
5. **What are the possible complications of drainage of acute parotitis or parotid abscess?**
   Possible complications of drainage of acute parotitis or parotid abscess include infection, bleeding, injury to the facial nerve, injury to surrounding structures (e.g. salivary ducts, blood vessels), and recurrence of parotitis or abscess.
6. **What are the anatomical landmarks of facial nerve main trunk in the parotid gland?**
   Pes anserinus: main trunk of facial nerve is identified by:
   Tragal pointer: facial nerve is 1 cm anterior, inferior, and deep (medial) to the tragal pointer.
   Tympano-mastoid suture: It is the most consistent and reliable landmark, and facial nerve is about 4–5 mm deep to the suture.
   Posterior belly of digastric muscle: as nerve lies in a plane deep to the muscle.

7. **What are the anatomical landmarks of main branches of facial nerve in the face?**

    Marginal mandibular nerve is about 1–2 mm below the angle of the mandible.

    Zygomatic: crosses zygomatic arch at its midpoint of a line between the tragus and lateral palpebral fissure.

    Buccal: 1 cm inferior and parallel to the parotid duct (Stensen duct line is located at the point midway between tragus and antitragus to a point at half upper lip).

6.13 Management of Traumatic Auricular Hematoma

Indications for Surgery

- Acute auricular haematoma causing pain and swelling.
- Risk of cartilage necrosis and subsequent cauliflower ear deformity.
- Recurrent or chronic auricular haematoma.

Specific Risks Involved with the Surgery

- Infection
- Bleeding
- Recurrence of haematoma
- Injury to the auricle or surrounding structures
- Suboptimal cosmetic result

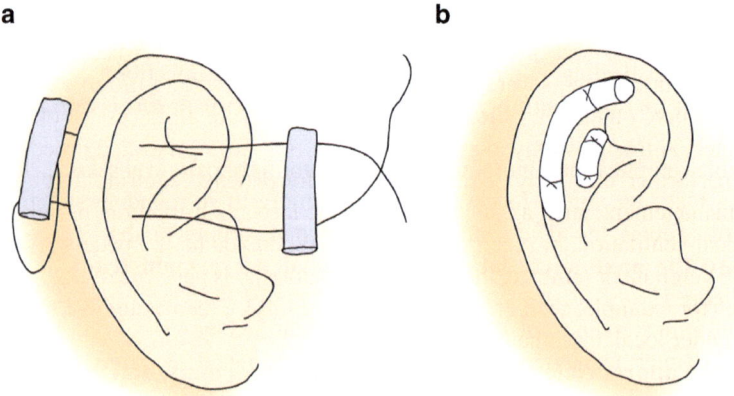

Fig. 6.14 Dental rolls sutured into pinna to apply pressure on incision site where a haematoma has been drained. (**a**) showing suture placed through dental rolls; (**b**) showing dental rolls compressing pinna haematoma. Illustrated by Vikum Liyanaarachchi

Steps of the Surgery

1. Preoperative assessment: Evaluate the patient's clinical condition, and determine the extent of the haematoma.
2. Anaesthesia: Administer local anaesthesia with or without sedation, depending on the patient's condition and the extent of the surgery. Perform a local anaesthetic ear block if required.
3. Incision: Make a small incision over the most prominent part of the haematoma, avoiding visible skin creases if possible.
4. Evacuation: Aspirate the haematoma using a syringe or gently express the clot with manual pressure.
5. Haemostasis: Achieve haemostasis using electrocautery or manual pressure as needed.
6. Placement of bolster dressing: Apply a non-adherent dressing to the incision site, and place a bolster dressing over the auricle to provide compression and prevent re-accumulation of the haematoma. For example, two dental rolls can be sutured onto the pinna as seen in Fig. 6.14.
7. Post-operative care: Instruct the patient to keep the area clean and dry, and monitor for any signs of infection, recurrent haematoma, or other complications.

Important Points to Note During the Surgery

- Prompt intervention is crucial to prevent cartilage necrosis and the development of cauliflower ear deformity.
- Ensure adequate haemostasis to minimize the risk of recurrent haematoma.
- Even pressure distribution with a bolster dressing is essential to prevent re-accumulation of the haematoma and to maintain the auricular shape.

Questions a Consultant Might Ask a Trainee About the Operation

1. **What is the primary goal of managing traumatic auricular haematoma?**
   The primary goal is to evacuate the haematoma, prevent its re-accumulation, and minimize the risk of cartilage necrosis and subsequent cauliflower ear deformity.
2. **What factors can increase the risk of complications following the management of a traumatic auricular haematoma?**
   Factors that can increase the risk of complications include delayed intervention, inadequate haemostasis, and uneven pressure distribution with the bolster dressing.
3. **How long should the bolster dressing be left in place following the surgery?**
   The bolster dressing should typically be left in place for 5–7 days to ensure proper healing and prevent re-accumulation of the haematoma.

4. **What are the possible complications of surgical management of traumatic auricular haematoma?**

    Possible complications include infection, bleeding, recurrence of haematoma, injury to the auricle or surrounding structures, and suboptimal cosmetic result, necrosis from the tight compression with auricular deformity.

5. **What measures can be taken to prevent recurrent auricular haematoma?**

    Measures to prevent recurrent auricular haematoma include achieving adequate haemostasis during surgery, applying even pressure with a bolster dressing, and avoiding activities that could cause further trauma to the ear.

6.14 Emergency Ligation of External Carotid Artery

Indications for Surgery

- Uncontrolled, life-threatening head and neck haemorrhage.
- Inability to control bleeding by other means (e.g. direct pressure, packing, endovascular techniques).

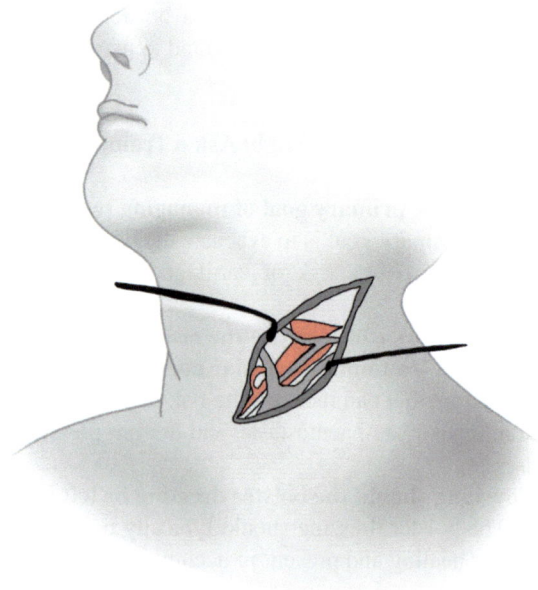

Fig. 6.15 Incision along SCM for identification of external carotid artery. Illustrated by Vikum Liyanaarachchi

Specific Risks Involved with the Surgery

- Infection
- Haematoma
- Injury to surrounding nerves or vessels
- Ischaemia of the supplied area
- Stroke (rare)

Steps of the Surgery

1. Preoperative assessment: Evaluate the patient's haemodynamic status, identify the source of the haemorrhage, and consider other treatment options.
2. Anaesthesia: Administer general anaesthesia with endotracheal intubation.
3. Positioning: Place the patient in a supine position with the neck extended and the head turned away from the side of the surgery.
4. Incision: Make a skin incision parallel to the anterior border of the sternocleidomastoid muscle, starting at the level of the thyroid cartilage and extending inferiorly towards the clavicle as seen in Fig. 6.15.
5. Dissection: Carefully dissect through the platysma and cervical fascia to expose the carotid sheath, taking care to avoid injury to the accessory nerve and other structures.
6. Identification: Identify the common carotid artery, and follow it superiorly to locate the bifurcation into the internal and external carotid arteries.
7. Isolation: Carefully isolate the external carotid artery from the surrounding structures, using vessel loops or ties for control.
8. Ensure that you have identified the external carotid artery correctly by identifying two or more branches (i.e. superior thyroid artery, lingual).
9. Ligation: Double ligate the external carotid artery using non-absorbable sutures, and then transect it between the ligatures if required. You may decide to ligate and not transect.
10. Haemostasis: Confirm haemostasis, and close any potential bleeding points.
11. Closure: Close the wound in layers, using absorbable sutures for the fascia and platysma and non-absorbable sutures or staples for the skin.

Important Points to Note During the Surgery

- Consider alternative treatments (e.g. endovascular techniques) if feasible and available.
- Carefully identify and preserve surrounding structures, such as nerves and vessels, during dissection.
- Ensure adequate haemostasis to minimize the risk of post-operative haematoma.

Questions a Consultant Might Ask a Trainee About the Operation

1. **What are the indications for emergency ligation of the external carotid artery?**
   The indications include uncontrolled, life-threatening head and neck haemorrhage and the inability to control bleeding by other means.
2. **What are the potential complications of this surgery?**
   Potential complications include infection, haematoma, injury to surrounding nerves or vessels, ischaemia of the supplied area, and stroke (rare).
3. **What are some alternative treatments to control life-threatening head and neck haemorrhage?**
   Alternative treatments include direct pressure, packing, and endovascular techniques such as embolization.
4. **How can the risk of injury to surrounding structures be minimized during this surgery?**
   Careful identification and preservation of surrounding structures, including nerves and vessels, during dissection can help minimize the risk of injury.
5. **How should the external carotid artery be ligated and transected during the surgery?**
   The external carotid artery should be double ligated using non-absorbable sutures and then transected between the ligatures.

6.15 Urgent Intervention for Airway Foreign Body (Ventilating Bronchoscopy or Oesophagoscopy)

Indications for Surgery

- Suspected foreign body in the airway causing respiratory distress or failure.
- Inability to remove the foreign body using basic airway manoeuvres (e.g. back blows, abdominal thrusts).

Specific Risks Involved with the Surgery

- Aspiration
- Laryngeal or tracheal injury
- Oesophageal perforation
- Bleeding
- Hypoxia

Steps of the Surgery

1. Preoperative assessment: Assess the patient's airway, breathing, and circulation, and obtain a history to determine the likelihood of a foreign body.

6 Emergencies

2. Anaesthesia: Administer general anaesthesia with spontaneous ventilation, avoiding muscle relaxants to maintain airway tone.
3. Patient positioning: Place the patient in a supine position with a shoulder roll to extend the neck.
4. Ventilating bronchoscopy: (a) Insert a bronchoscope into the patient's mouth, and advance it through the vocal cords into the trachea. (b) Inspect the trachea and bronchi, looking for the foreign body. (c) Use forceps or suction to grasp and remove the foreign body. See Fig. 6.7 for a diagram of the bronchoscope.
5. Oesophagoscopy: (a) Insert an oesophagoscope into the patient's mouth, and advance it into the oesophagus. (b) Inspect the oesophagus, looking for the foreign body. (c) Use forceps to grasp and remove the foreign body.
6. Post-removal: Perform a thorough inspection of the airway or oesophagus to ensure no residual fragments or injuries.
7. Recovery: Monitor the patient's airway, breathing, and circulation, and provide appropriate post-operative care.

Important Points to Note During the Surgery

- Maintain spontaneous ventilation to preserve airway tone and minimize the risk of dislodging the foreign body.
- Be prepared to manage potential complications, such as aspiration or bleeding.
- Use gentle force and appropriate instruments to minimize the risk of injury to the airway or oesophagus.
- After removal of the foreign body, a second look is needed to make sure that there is no other foreign body or residual.

Questions a Consultant Might Ask a Trainee About the Operation

1. **What are some common foreign bodies encountered in the airway, and how might the presentation vary based on the location of the foreign body?**
   Common foreign bodies include food particles (e.g. nuts, seeds), small toys, and dental appliances. The presentation may vary based on the location of the foreign body. For instance, a foreign body in the larynx may cause stridor and hoarseness, while one in the bronchus may present with localized wheezing or decreased breath sounds.
2. **How can you differentiate between a foreign body lodged in the airway and one lodged in the oesophagus based on clinical presentation?**
   A foreign body in the airway typically presents with respiratory symptoms such as coughing, choking, stridor, or wheezing, while a foreign body in the oesophagus may cause dysphagia, odynophagia, or drooling. However, the presentations can overlap, and diagnostic imaging or endoscopy may be required to confirm the location of the foreign body.

3. **In cases where a foreign body is lodged in the airway and cannot be immediately removed, what other interventions can be considered to temporarily maintain airway patency?**

   If a foreign body cannot be immediately removed, other interventions to maintain airway patency may include the use of a supraglottic airway device, endotracheal intubation, or, in extreme cases, an emergency cricothyroidotomy or tracheostomy.

4. **What factors should be considered when deciding between a rigid and a flexible bronchoscope for airway foreign body removal?**

   The choice between a rigid and flexible bronchoscope depends on factors such as the patient's age, size, and anatomy, as well as the size, location, and composition of the foreign body. A rigid bronchoscope offers better visualization and larger working channels for instrument use but may be less suitable for small children or patients with difficult airway anatomy. A flexible bronchoscope is less invasive and can navigate more distal airways but may have limitations in visualization and instrument use.

5. **What is the role of diagnostic imaging in the management of suspected airway foreign bodies, and what imaging modalities are commonly used?**

   Diagnostic imaging can help confirm the presence and location of a foreign body, as well as evaluate for complications such as pneumothorax or mediastinal emphysema. Common imaging modalities include plain radiography (e.g. anteroposterior and lateral neck, chest, or abdominal X-rays) and computed tomography (CT). Radiolucent foreign bodies may be more challenging to visualize, and the clinical presentation may guide the choice of imaging.

6. **What type of bronchoscope can be used to aid in visualization of the FB?**

   Right ventilating bronchoscope with optical grasping forceps. Adrenaline 1:10,000 could be used and injected through the suction port to aid in decongestant and improve visualization.

7. **What anaesthetic technique is preferred in the removal of foreign body from the airway?**

   Spontaneous ventilation is preferable. It is recommended to maintain spontaneous breathing or gentle assisted ventilation as positive pressure may dislodge the foreign body further distally.

   Sevoflurane in 100% oxygen and topical anaesthesia to the airway are the techniques of choice. Total intravenous anaesthesia can also be used.

8. **Do you know any charts for identifying the size of the tracheostomy tube, endotracheal tube, or bronchoscopy size?**

   Great Ormond Street Hospital (GOSH) Chart for Paediatric Airway

6.16 Urgent Management of Penetrating Neck Trauma

Indications for Surgery

- Active haemorrhage or expanding haematoma
- Haemodynamic instability

- Airway compromise
- Vascular injury (e.g. stroke symptoms, bruit, or thrill)
- Aerodigestive tract injury (e.g. subcutaneous emphysema, haematemesis, or haemoptysis)

Specific Risks Involved with the Surgery

- Damage to adjacent structures (e.g. nerves, vessels, trachea, or oesophagus)
- Infection
- Bleeding or haematoma formation
- Air embolism
- Pneumothorax or pneumomediastinum

Steps of the Surgery

1. Secure the airway, if needed (e.g. endotracheal intubation, cricothyroidotomy, or tracheostomy).
2. Establish intravenous access, and initiate fluid resuscitation.
3. Assess the patient's haemodynamic status and neurological function.
4. Expose and explore the neck wound, taking care to identify and protect vital structures.
5. Control active bleeding using direct pressure, electrocautery, or vascular clamps.
6. Repair injured vessels using sutures or vascular grafts.
7. Inspect the aerodigestive tract for injuries and repair as needed (e.g. primary closure, stenting, or diversion).
8. Perform a thorough debridement of the wound, and irrigate with saline.
9. Perform panendoscopy with rigid oesophagoscopy also to ensure no other injuries.
10. Close the wound in layers with appropriate sutures.
11. Monitor the patient closely in the post-operative period for signs of complications.

Important Points to Note During the Surgery

- Consider the anatomical zones of the neck (I, II, and III) to guide surgical exploration and management.
- Be prepared to address airway and haemodynamic emergencies.
- Work closely with a multidisciplinary team, including vascular, trauma, and thoracic surgeons, as needed.
- Perform a thorough evaluation of the neck, including vascular and aerodigestive structures.
- Consider the need for diagnostic imaging, such as CT angiography, to assess for vascular injuries.

Questions a Consultant Might Ask a Trainee About the Operation

1. **What are the anatomical zones of the neck, and how do they influence the management of penetrating neck trauma?**
   The neck is divided into three zones:
   Zone I extends from the clavicle to the cricoid cartilage; Zone II is from the cricoid cartilage to the angle of the mandible; and Zone III is from the angle of the mandible to the skull base. Injuries in Zone II are more easily accessible and can often be explored directly, whereas Zone I and Zone III injuries may require further diagnostic imaging and a multidisciplinary approach.
2. **What are some of the most common vascular injuries seen in penetrating neck trauma?**
   Common vascular injuries include injuries to the carotid artery, internal jugular vein, vertebral artery, and subclavian vessels.
3. **How can you differentiate between tracheal and oesophageal injuries in the setting of penetrating neck trauma?**
   Tracheal injuries may present with subcutaneous emphysema, dyspnoea, or pneumothorax, while oesophageal injuries may present with haematemesis, dysphagia, or odynophagia. Direct visualization and endoscopic evaluation can help confirm the diagnosis.
4. **What are some potential complications of an undiagnosed or untreated aerodigestive injury following penetrating neck trauma?**
   Potential complications include infection (e.g. mediastinitis or abscess), fistula formation, sepsis, and airway compromise. Delayed diagnosis and treatment can lead to increased morbidity and mortality.
5. **In the setting of penetrating neck trauma, when is it appropriate to perform a selective neck exploration vs. a non-operative management approach?**
   Selective neck exploration is indicated in patients with "hard signs" of injury (e.g. active haemorrhage, expanding haematoma, airway compromise, vascular injury, or aerodigestive tract injury). Non-operative management, including close observation and possible further diagnostic imaging, may be appropriate for patients with "soft signs" of injury (e.g. stable haematoma, minor bleeding, or non-expanding subcutaneous emphysema) or no signs of injury, provided that there is a low suspicion of underlying injuries to vital structures.
6. **What are the signs of vascular injury?**
   The signs of vascular injury are critical for early diagnosis and management, including the following:
   - Inspection: An expanding haematoma or active bleeding from a wound suggests a significant vascular injury. Look for visible signs of blood pooling or an enlarging mass under the skin.
   - Palpation: A bruit (a whooshing sound heard over a blood vessel) or thrill (a palpable vibration) indicates an arteriovenous fistula. Check for coolness, pallor, or delayed capillary refill distal to the injury, which are signs of reduced blood flow or distal ischaemia.

- Auscultation: Absence of a pulse (pulselessness) or a weaker pulse compared to the opposite limb (pulse deficit) is an alarming sign of arterial occlusion or severe vascular compromise.

7. **What are the signs of airway injury?**

   Recognizing airway injury is paramount for preventing life-threatening complications:
   - Fibre-optic examination: This allows for the direct visualization of the internal structures of the airway, identifying disruptions, obstructions, or oedema that might not be externally visible.
   - Inspection: Stridor (a high-pitched wheezing sound), wheezing, or overt signs of respiratory distress (e.g. tachypnoea, use of accessory muscles for breathing, cyanosis) indicate a compromised airway.
   - Palpation: The presence of subcutaneous emphysema (air trapped under the skin) or laryngeal crepitus (crackling sensation over the larynx due to air in the soft tissues) around the neck, chest, or face signals an air leak from the respiratory tract, which could be due to a tear or puncture.

8. **Is Gastrografin swallow recommended in the management of oesophageal perforation?**

   Gastrografin swallow should be approached with caution in the context of oesophageal perforation due to the risk of exacerbating the injury or failing to detect certain types of damage. Initially, it is not recommended because of the potential for introducing contrast material into the mediastinum or pleural space, which can cause inflammation or infection. However, after 5–7 days post-injury or following surgical repair of the oesophagus, a Gastrografin swallow study can be useful for assessing the integrity of the repair and ensuring that there are no leaks.

9. **What is the Schaefer classification system for laryngeal trauma?**

   The Schaefer classification system categorizes laryngeal trauma into five groups based on the severity and treatment approach:
   - Groups 1 and 2: Represent minor to moderate injuries (e.g. haematomas, lacerations without exposed cartilage, minor mucosal disruptions, or nondisplaced fractures), often managed conservatively with observation and possibly steroids.
   - Groups 3 and 4: Indicate more severe injuries with significant structural damage (e.g. massive oedema, exposed cartilage, displaced fractures, vocal cord immobility), typically requiring surgical intervention, which might include tracheostomy for airway management and repair of the laryngeal framework.
   - Group 5: Denotes the most severe form of injury, complete laryngotracheal separation, requiring immediate and aggressive surgical intervention for reestablishment of the airway and reconstruction of the laryngeal framework.

10. **How should a tracheal tear be managed?**

    A tracheal tear represents a critical condition requiring prompt management to secure the airway and prevent further damage:

- Ventilating bronchoscope: Use for direct visualization of the tear, allowing for precise management and potentially aiding in the placement of a tracheal stent or guiding surgical repair.
- Flexible guided intubation: Employed to bypass the site of the tear and provide stable ventilation, ideally under the guidance of visualization tools to avoid exacerbating the injury.
- Tracheostomy: Considered when intubation is not feasible or might worsen the tear, providing a secure airway below the site of injury. It is essential to approach tracheostomy with care, particularly in the presence of subcutaneous emphysema, which can alter neck anatomy and increase the risk of complications.

References

1. Bonanno FG. Techniques for emergency tracheostomy. Injury. 2008;39(3):375–8.
2. McGrath BA, Bates L, Atkinson D, Moore JA. Multidisciplinary guidelines for the management of tracheostomy and laryngectomy airway emergencies. Anaesthesia. 2012;67(9):1025–41. https://doi.org/10.1111/j.1365-2044.2012.07217.x.
3. Frerk C, Mitchell VS, McNarry AF, et al. Difficult Airway Society 2015 guidelines for management of unanticipated difficult intubation in adults. Br J Anaesth. 2015;115(6):827–48. https://doi.org/10.1093/bja/aev371.
4. Schroeder AA. Cricothyroidotomy: when, why, and why not? Am J Otolaryngol. 2000;21(3):195–201.
5. Snyderman CH, Goldman SA, Carrau RL, Ferguson BJ, Grandis JR. Endoscopic sphenopalatine artery ligation is an effective method of treatment for posterior epistaxis. Am J Rhinol. 1999;13(2):137–40.
6. Taylor MF, Berkowitz RG. Indications for mastoidectomy in acute mastoiditis in children. Ann Otol Rhinol Laryngol. 2004;113(1):69–72.

Facial Plastics

Sami AlHassan, Zohaib Siddiqui, Basim Wahba, and Keli Dusu

7.1 Otoplasty

Indications for Surgery [1]

- Congenital ear deformities
  - Protruding ears
  - Aesthetic concerns related to the size, shape, or position of the ears
- Asymmetrical ears

Risks Involved with the Surgery [1]

- Bleeding
- Infection
- Scarring
- Nerve injury (e.g. sensory nerves)

Every procedure requires photodocumentation before and after.

S. AlHassan (✉)
The Royal London Hospital, London, UK
e-mail: sami.alhasan@nhs.net

Z. Siddiqui
Medway NHS Foundation Trust, Gillingham, Kent, UK

B. Wahba
Queen Victoria Hospital, East Grinstead, West Sussex, UK

K. Dusu
Frimley Park Hospital, Frimley, Camberley, UK

- Asymmetry or unsatisfactory cosmetic result
- Recurrence of the deformity
- Anaesthesia complications
- Cartilage necrosis
- Overcorrection/undercorrection
- Telephone and reverse telephone deformity
- Hearing loss due to narrowing of external ear canal and anteriorly placed Furnas sutures

Steps of the Surgery

1. Preoperative planning:
2. Detailed assessment:
   - Conduct a thorough evaluation of the patient's ear anatomy, focusing on the size, shape, and symmetry of the ears.
   - Pay special attention to the auriculocephalic angle (the angle between the ear and the head), the size of the conchal bowl, and the definition of the antihelical fold.
   - Discuss the patient's specific goals, such as reducing protrusion or correcting asymmetry, and manage expectations realistically.
   - Ensure that adequate photography is performed pre-op.
3. Marking Incision Sites:
   - Mark the areas on the posterior aspect of the ear where incisions will be made, usually within the natural crease to hide scars effectively.
   - Plan the extent of skin excision (if needed) and areas where cartilage will be modified.
4. Anaesthesia:
   - Apply local anaesthesia with or without sedation to numb the ear area. This is often sufficient for adult patients.
   - In children or for patients who prefer, general anaesthesia can be administered for added comfort and immobility during the procedure.
5. Incision:
   - Perform a posterior incision along the pre-marked lines behind the ear. This incision provides access to the ear cartilage while concealing the scar.
   - Carefully incise through the skin and superficial tissues to expose the underlying cartilage.
6. Elevating Skin and Soft Tissues:
   - Gently elevate the skin and soft tissues off the cartilage, preserving as much of the perichondrium (the connective tissue layer covering the cartilage) as possible to maintain blood supply and support healing.
7. Cartilage Reshaping:
   - Score the cartilage on its anterior surface to weaken it, and create a more defined antihelical fold.
   - Excise a portion of the cartilage, particularly in the conchal bowl area, to reduce ear protrusion.

- Suturing techniques (like Mustarde or Furnas sutures) are used to fold the cartilage and create or enhance the antihelical fold. See Fig. 7.1 for an example.
8. Suture Fixation:
    - Use non-absorbable sutures to fix the cartilage in its new position, ensuring that the ear lies closer to the head at the desired angle.
    - Place sutures carefully to avoid altering the natural ear contours or creating sharp edges.

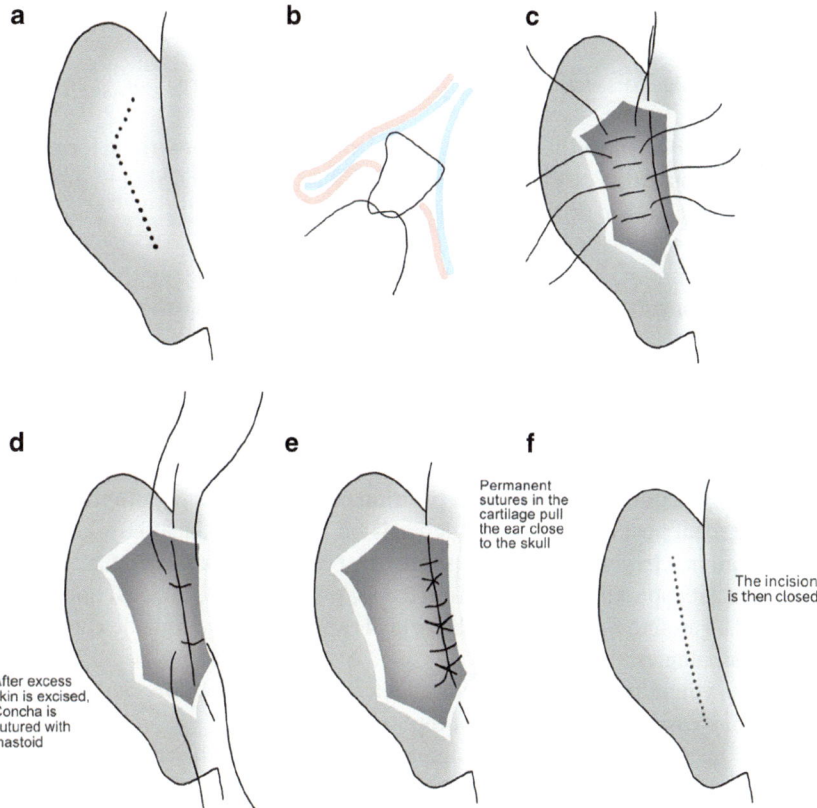

Fig. 7.1 Example of the Furnas suture for otoplasty. (**a**) **Initial incision marks**: Dotted lines indicate where the incision will be made behind the ear, outlining the area for the surgical approach. (**b**) **Cartilage and anatomy overview**: Diagram showing the anatomical structures involved in the surgery, including the conchal cartilage and adjacent tissues. (**c**) **Conchal cartilage exposure**: The skin is incised, and the conchal cartilage is exposed to prepare for suturing. (**d**) **Excess skin removal and suturing preparation**: Excess skin is excised, and the conchal cartilage is prepared for suturing to the mastoid. (**e**) **Placement of permanent sutures**: Permanent sutures are placed in the cartilage, pulling the ear closer to the skull and securing the new position of the ear. (**f**) **Incision closure**: The surgical incision is closed with sutures, completing the Furnas suture technique for otoplasty. Illustrated by Vikum Liyanaarachchi

9. Closure:
    - Suture the posterior incision meticulously with absorbable or non-absorbable sutures, ensuring proper alignment of the wound edges for minimal scarring.
    - Apply a light dressing to protect the site.
    - Place a compressive headband over the ears to support the new position and reduce post-operative swelling. This headband is typically worn for 24 h. Following this, it is advised the patient wears a headband for 1 week every day/night and then only at night for 1 month.

Important Points to Note During the Surgery

- Use meticulous dissection techniques to minimize the risk of scarring or nerve injury.
- Ensure proper haemostasis to reduce the risk of haematoma or seroma formation.
- Avoid overcorrection or excessive tension on the cartilage and skin to minimize the risk of recurrence or unsatisfactory cosmetic results.

Questions a Consultant Might Ask a Trainee About the Operation

1. **What are the key anatomical landmarks to consider during otoplasty?**
    Key landmarks include the conchal bowl, antihelix, helical rim, and scapha. Proper identification and manipulation of these structures are crucial for achieving a natural and aesthetically pleasing result.
2. **How do you determine the ideal position of the ears during otoplasty?**
    The ideal position of the ears depends on the patient's anatomy, goals, and expectations. In general, the ears should be positioned parallel to the temporal line and sit approximately 2 cm from the mastoid skin. The conchal bowl depth should be around 1–1.5 cm, and the helical rim should have a gentle curve without sharp angles.
3. **How do you manage complications such as haematoma, infection, or unsatisfactory cosmetic results after otoplasty?**
    For haematomas, prompt recognition and management are crucial. Small haematomas may be managed conservatively with compression and close observation, while larger ones may require surgical evacuation and exploration to identify and control any bleeding sources. Infections should be treated with appropriate antibiotics and may require drainage if an abscess is present. Unsatisfactory cosmetic results may be addressed through revision surgery, considering the specific concerns and patient goals.
4. **What are the advantages and disadvantages of using scoring, excision, or suturing techniques for cartilage reshaping during otoplasty?**
    Scoring techniques weaken the cartilage to allow for reshaping but may result in visible irregularities or sharp angles. Excision techniques remove excess cartilage but can result in overcorrection or loss of natural contours.

Suturing techniques can achieve more precise reshaping and positioning but may be more technically challenging.

5. **What is the role of a compressive headband after otoplasty?**
   A compressive headband helps to stabilize the ear in its new position, minimize swelling, and protect the ears from inadvertent trauma.

6. **What is the preferred age in which to perform otoplasty in children?**
   Most surgeons will wait until the age of at least 6 years of age, as the auricle is then 90–95% of adult size. It can be done under 6 years of age if required due to bullying or if a hearing aid is required.

7. **What are the features of prominent ears?**
   Presence of one or a combination of obtuse antihelix–deep conchal bowl–increased mastoid-helix angle to more than >30 degrees with anterior rotation. A normal ear is described as one that has a mastoid-helix angle of 20 degrees.

8. **What is the Frankfurt line?**
   From the top of the porion (upper margin of external auditory canal) till the lower border of lower orbital rim). In otoplasty, the distance of auricle to mastoid at Frankfurt line is normally 15–18 mm.

9. **Are there any non-surgical options available for the patient/family to consider?**
   Taping the Auricle to the Head: This method involves gently taping the affected ear(s) closer to the head to encourage them to grow in a more typical position. It is a simple and non-invasive technique that can be effective, especially in newborns and young infants, whose ear cartilage is still very soft and flexible. This method can sometimes be sufficient for mild cases of ear deformity, such as protruding ears.

   Malleable Splints (e.g. Ear Buddies): Ear splints are another non-surgical option that can be used to correct ear deformities. Products like Ear Buddies are designed to reshape the soft cartilage of the ears, guiding them into a more typical shape and position. The splints are taped to the pinna (the visible part of the ear) and can be worn continuously for several weeks. Because the cartilage in infants' ears is most pliable in the first few weeks of life, this method is particularly effective in newborns and infants.

10. **What are the surgical options? What are the common suture techniques?**
    Cartilage-Sparing Techniques
    - These techniques aim to reshape the ear without removing or significantly altering the cartilage.
    - Mustarde technique: This method uses sutures to correct the fold of the ear (the antihelix) when it is not well defined. Concho-scaphoid sutures are placed to create or enhance the antihelical fold, thus reducing the prominence of the ear.
    - Furnas technique: This involves placing sutures between the concha (the deep bowl-like part of the external ear) and the mastoid process (the bony area behind the ear) to pull the ear back closer to the head, addressing issues with excessive conchal bowl prominence.

    Cartilage Non-sparing Techniques
    - These approaches involve more direct alteration of the ear cartilage.

- Incision scoring (Stenstrom technique): This method involves making incisions on the cartilage and then scoring (scratching or cutting into) the cartilage to encourage it to bend or fold in a desired way, thus changing the ear's shape.
- Incision suturing (converse technique): Similar to the Mustarde technique, it involves reshaping the ear through strategic suturing but includes making incisions to facilitate the reshaping process.
- Cartilage thinning (Weerda technique): This technique involves thinning the cartilage with a burring tool to make it more pliable and easier to reshape. It is often used in combination with other techniques to achieve the desired ear contour.
- Minimally Invasive Options
- Ear-fold implants: This is a more recent, minimally invasive option where small incisions are made to create pockets for the implantation of ear-fold implants. These implants are designed to correct the prominence of the ears by creating or enhancing the antihelical fold, offering a less invasive alternative to traditional surgery.
- Suture Techniques
- Mustarde's concho-scaphoid sutures: Used to create or enhance the antihelical fold by bringing the scapha closer to the conchal bowl.
- Furnas' concho-mastoid sutures: Aimed at reducing the angle between the ear and the side of the head by securing the concha to the mastoid process.
- *The techniques can also be divided as incision and incision-less.*

11. **What type of suture, needle, and suturing technique you would use with Mustarde?**

    Suture: 4-0 non-absorbable suture: A 4-0 gauge non-absorbable suture is commonly used. Non-absorbable sutures are preferred for their durability and strength, as they need to maintain the ear's new shape permanently. The thickness of the suture (4-0) strikes a balance between being strong enough to hold the cartilage in place and thin enough to minimize scarring and discomfort.

    Needle: Inverted cutting needle: An inverted cutting needle is designed to cut through tissue with minimal resistance and is less likely to shear or damage the cartilage compared to other needle types. Its cutting edge is on the inner curvature of the needle, which allows for precise placement of sutures without causing unnecessary trauma to the cartilage.

    Suturing technique: Horizontal mattress suturing: This technique involves placing sutures in a way that they loop around the cartilage, pulling it into the desired shape without cutting through it. The horizontal mattress suturing technique is effective for reshaping the ear because it distributes tension evenly, reduces the risk of suture cut-through, and promotes a more natural-looking fold in the antihelix.

    Implementation: During the procedure, the surgeon makes precise incisions behind the ear to expose the cartilage. The 4-0 non-absorbable sutures are then placed using the inverted cutting needle, applying the horizontal mattress suturing technique to fold and secure the cartilage into the desired new shape.

7 Facial Plastics

The placement and tension of the sutures are critical for achieving a natural-looking antihelical fold and ensuring that the ear lies closer to the head.

7.2 Skin Cancer Excisions and Reconstruction

Indications for Surgery

- Skin cancer diagnosis (e.g. basal cell carcinoma, squamous cell carcinoma, melanoma)
- Aesthetic or functional concerns related to skin cancer or its treatment

Specific Risks Involved with the Surgery

- Bleeding
- Infection
- Scarring—keloid
- Nerve injury—numbness (otherwise depending on location)
- Recurrence of skin cancer
- Anaesthesia complications
- Graft failure/necrosis

Steps of the Surgery

1. Preoperative planning: Assess the location, size, and characteristics of the skin cancer. Plan the excision margins based on the type and stage of cancer, as well as the reconstruction technique, considering the size and location of the defect, patient's anatomy, and goals.
2. Anaesthesia: Administer local anaesthesia with or without sedation, depending on patient preference and medical factors.
3. Marking: Outline the skin cancer and planned excision margins with a surgical marker. Design the incision and reconstruction to optimize functional and aesthetic outcomes.
4. Excision:
   (a) Incise the skin along the marked excision margins, using a scalpel or electrocautery.
   (b) Perform careful dissection around the tumour, ensuring complete removal while preserving vital structures such as nerves and blood vessels.
   (c) Excise the skin cancer with appropriate margins, and send the specimen for histopathological analysis to confirm clear margins.
5. Haemostasis: Ensure proper haemostasis by using electrocautery or suture ligatures to control bleeding.

6. Reconstruction: (a) Assess the defect, and select the appropriate reconstruction technique based on the reconstruction ladder. (b) Prepare the recipient site by debriding non-viable tissue and ensuring adequate blood supply. (c) Perform the chosen reconstruction technique, which may include primary closure, secondary intention healing, skin grafts, local flaps, or regional or free flaps. (d) If using a skin graft, harvest the graft from the donor site, and secure it to the recipient site using sutures or staples. (e) If using a flap, design and elevate the flap, then transpose, rotate, or advance it to cover the defect, ensuring proper positioning and tension-free closure.
7. Closure: Close the incision with sutures, ensuring good apposition of the wound edges and tension-free closure. Apply a light dressing.
8. Post-operative care: Provide instructions for wound care, pain management, and follow-up visits to monitor healing and address any concerns.

Important Points to Note During the Surgery

- Ensure complete removal of the skin cancer with appropriate margins to minimize the risk of recurrence.
- Choose the appropriate reconstruction technique based on the size, location, and characteristics of the defect, as well as the patient's goals and expectations.
- Preserve the integrity of surrounding nerves and blood vessels to minimize the risk of nerve injury or bleeding.

Reconstruction Ladder

The reconstruction ladder (Fig. 7.2) is a stepwise approach to reconstructing defects after skin cancer excision. The main options, in increasing order of complexity, include:

1. Secondary intention healing: Allowing the wound to heal naturally by granulation tissue formation. Suitable for small defects in areas with good blood supply and low tension.
2. Primary closure: Direct closure of the wound edges with sutures. Suitable for small, uncomplicated defects.
3. Skin grafts: Harvesting skin from a donor site and placing it on the defect. Split-thickness skin grafts include the epidermis and part of the dermis, while full-thickness grafts include both layers. Suitable for larger defects without significant depth or complex contouring.
4. Local flaps: Using adjacent tissue to cover the defect. Techniques include advancement flaps, rotation flaps, and transposition flaps (Fig. 7.3). Suitable for defects requiring more complex contouring or when primary closure is not possible due to tension.
5. Regional or free flaps: Transferring tissue from a distant site to cover the defect, either with an intact blood supply (regional flaps) or with microvascular anastomosis (free flaps). Suitable for large, complex defects or when local flaps are not possible or insufficient.

Fig. 7.2 An example of the reconstructive ladder used for repair. Illustrated by Vikum Liyanaarachchi

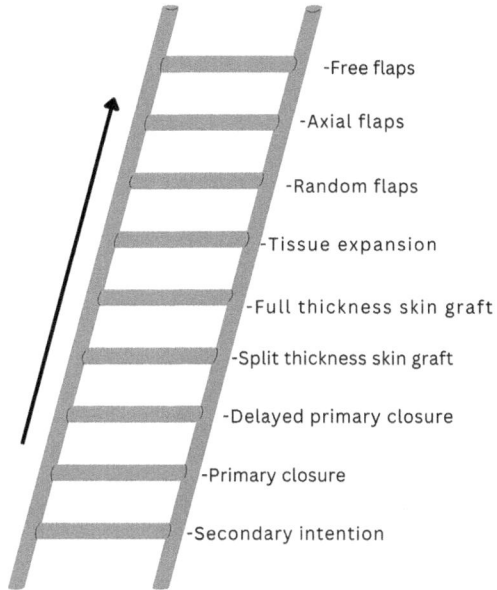

Questions a Consultant Might Ask a Trainee About the Operation

1. **How do you determine the appropriate excision margins for different types of skin cancer?**

   Excision margins depend on the type and stage of skin cancer. For example, basal cell carcinoma typically requires 4–5 mm margins, while squamous cell carcinoma may require 4–6 mm margins, and melanoma margins depend on the tumour thickness [2].

2. **What factors should be considered when selecting a reconstruction technique after skin cancer excision?**

   Factors to consider include the size, location, and characteristics of the defect; patient's goals and expectations; and the surgeon's experience and preference. The reconstruction ladder provides a stepwise approach to guide the selection process.

3. **How do you manage complications such as infection, flap necrosis, or unsatisfactory cosmetic results after skin cancer excision and reconstruction?**

   Infections should be managed with appropriate antibiotics, and, in some cases, wound debridement or drainage may be necessary. Flap necrosis can be addressed through revision surgery, which may involve debridement of non-viable tissue and re-evaluation of the reconstruction technique. Unsatisfactory cosmetic results may require additional procedures to address specific concerns and patient goals, such as scar revision, further excision, or alternative reconstruction techniques.

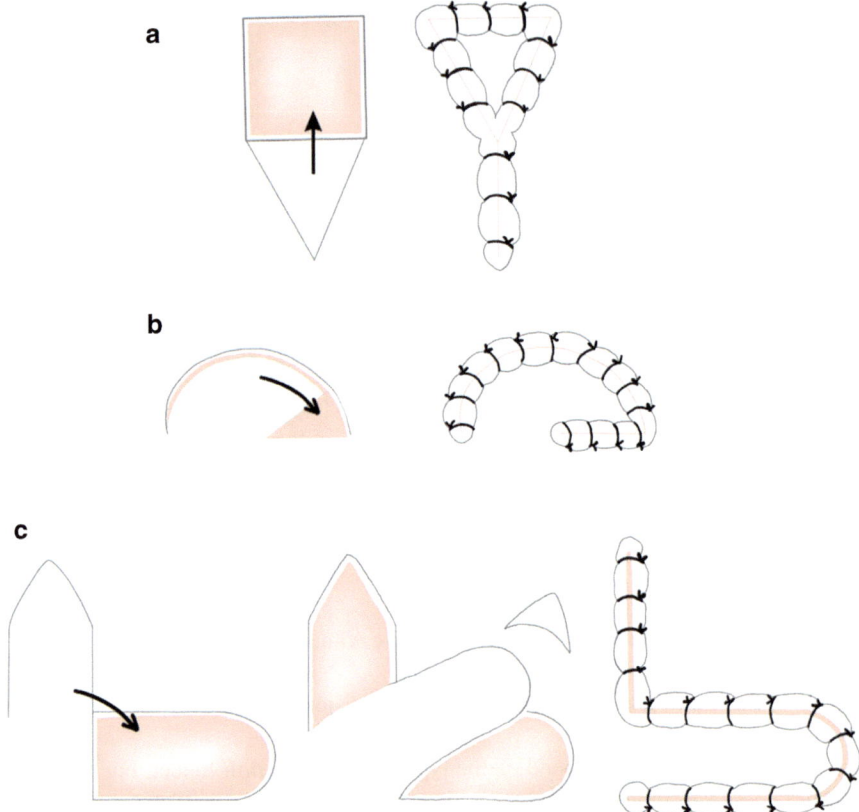

Fig. 7.3 Examples of local skin flaps. (**a**) V-Y Advancement Flap: This example illustrates a V-Y advancement flap, where a V-shaped incision is made, and the flap is advanced forward to close a defect. The arms of the "V" are then sutured together in a "Y" configuration, allowing for direct advancement of the tissue without significant rotation. This technique is often used to close small defects with minimal tension. (**b**) Rotation Flap: This example shows a rotation flap, where a semicircular incision allows for the rotation of a skin flap to cover an adjacent defect. The arrow indicates the direction of rotation, providing coverage with nearby tissue while minimizing tension at the closure site. (**c**) Transposition Flap: This illustration depicts a transposition flap, where skin from an adjacent area is lifted and moved into the defect. The flap is then sutured into place, allowing for closure with tissue that is similar in texture and thickness to the original defect site. The arrow shows the direction of movement. Illustrated by Vikum Liyanaarachchi

4. **How do you minimize the risk of nerve injury during skin cancer excision and reconstruction?**

    To minimize nerve injury, identify and preserve the nerves during dissection, use blunt dissection techniques, and ensure that the reconstruction does not apply excessive pressure on the nerves. Proper patient selection and preoperative planning can also help minimize the risk of nerve injury.

5. **How do you manage the donor site after harvesting a skin graft or flap?**

   Management of the donor site depends on the type of graft or flap harvested. For split-thickness skin grafts, the donor site may be dressed with a non-adherent dressing and allowed to heal by secondary intention. For full-thickness skin grafts and local flaps, the donor site may be closed primarily with sutures. In the case of regional or free flaps, the donor site may require a separate skin graft or closure technique to achieve optimal healing and minimize complications. Proper donor site care is essential to prevent infection, bleeding, and poor healing.

6. **In primary closure of surgical or traumatic wounds, how much can undermining typically extend the closure capacity?**

   Undermining can often extend the closure capacity up to four times the width of the original defect.

7. **When reconstructing facial lesions, which principles are essential to follow?**

   Ensuring that the axis of the scar aligns with the relaxed skin tension lines (RSTLs) or falls within the margin of the subunit is crucial.

   It is also important to consider the involvement of facial subunits; if more than 50% of a subunit is affected, replacing the entire unit is advised.

8. **What constitutes the facial units?**

   The face is divided into five main units: forehead, eye, nose, cheek, and lips and chin, each comprising multiple subunits.

9. **What benefits does a full-thickness skin graft (FTSG), also known as a Wolfe graft, have over a split-thickness skin graft (STSG)?**

   An FTSG generally offers a better cosmetic outcome, featuring colour and texture that more closely match the surrounding skin when harvested from areas like the pre/postauricular or supraclavicular regions for facial defects. It is thicker, more durable, and less prone to contracture than an STSG, though it carries a higher risk of graft failure.

10. **What criteria classify skin basal cell carcinoma (BCC) as high risk, necessitating removal with margins exceeding 5 mm, according to the British Association of Dermatology Guidelines?**

    Tumours larger than 2 cm, located in complex areas such as the central face, exhibiting high-risk histology types (morphic, micronodular pigmented, basosquamous), with poorly defined margins, perivascular or perineural invasion, recurrence, and cases involving immunosuppressed patients are deemed high risk.

11. **What criteria define high-risk squamous cell carcinoma (SCC) of the skin?**

    SCC is considered high risk if the tumour size exceeds 2 cm or has a depth of invasion >2 mm, is in the ear or on a hair-bearing lip, shows high-risk histology types (poorly differentiated or undifferentiated), involves perivascular or perineural invasion, has recurred, or occurs in immunosuppressed patients.

    Low-risk lesions should be excised with at least a 4–6 mm margin, whereas high-risk and very-high-risk lesions require excision with a margin of 6 mm or 10 mm, respectively.

7.3 Scar Revision

Indications for Surgery

- Hypertrophic or keloid scars
- Scars causing functional impairment (e.g. contractures)
- Scars causing aesthetic concerns or disfigurement

Risks Involved with the Surgery

- Bleeding
- Infection
- Recurrence or worsening of the scar

Steps of the Surgery

1. Preoperative planning: Assess the scar's location, size, and characteristics. Plan the incision and revision technique.
2. Anaesthesia: Administer local anaesthesia with or without sedation, depending on patient preference and medical factors.
3. Incision: Excise the scar tissue using an appropriate technique, such as elliptical excision, W-plasty, Z-plasty (Fig. 7.4), or geometric broken line closure.
4. Closure: Close the incision with sutures, ensuring good apposition of the wound edges and tension-free closure. Apply a light dressing.
5. Post-operative care: Instruct the patient on proper wound care, and consider adjunctive therapies such as silicone gel sheeting, pressure garments, or corticosteroid injections to optimize the final scar appearance.

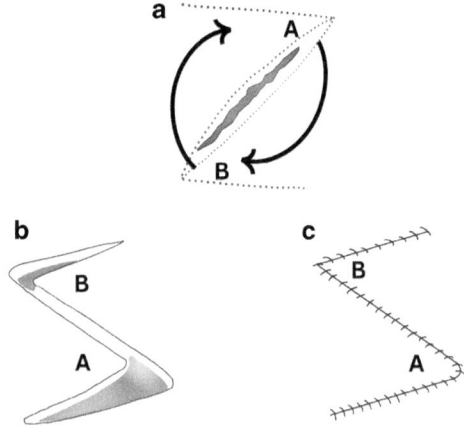

Fig. 7.4 Example of Z-plasty. (**a**) **Incision planning**: Mark Z-shaped incisions with arms A and B. Arrows show flap transposition direction. (**b**) **Flap creation**: Make incisions along marked lines to create triangular flaps A and B. (**c**) **Transposition and suturing**: Transpose flaps A and B, securing them with sutures in their new positions. Illustrated by Vikum Liyanaarachchi

Important Points to Note During the Surgery

- Preserve the integrity of surrounding nerves and blood vessels to minimize the risk of nerve injury or bleeding.
- Ensure proper suturing and tension-free closure to promote optimal wound healing and minimize scar recurrence.
- Keep note of Langer's lines (lines of skin tension) when creating any incision to aid aesthetic results.
- Dermal fat graft, dermabrasion, laser treatment, and fillers are options for surface treatment to improve scar appearance.

Questions a Consultant Might Ask a Trainee About the Operation

1. **Name the different classifications of scars.**
   Scars can be classified into five main types: keloid scars, contracted scars, rolling scars, hypertrophic scars, and atrophic scars.
2. **What are the key principles of scar revision surgery?**
   Key principles include excision of the scar tissue, proper tissue handling, tension-free closure, removal of any foreign bodies or necrotic tissues, closure with least reactive suture material, and appropriate post-operative care to optimize the final scar appearance and minimize recurrence.
3. **How do you decide between different scar revision techniques (e.g. W-plasty, Z-plasty, geometric broken line closure)?**
   The choice of technique depends on the scar's location, size, and characteristics, as well as the surgeon's experience and preference. W-plasty and Z-plasty can help break up linear scars and redistribute tension, while geometric broken line closure can make the scar less noticeable by blending it with the surrounding skin's natural contours.
4. **What adjunctive therapies can be used to optimize scar appearance after scar revision surgery?**
   Adjunctive therapies include silicone gel sheeting, pressure garments, and corticosteroid injections. These therapies can help reduce scar thickness, discoloration, and itching, promoting a better final appearance. The choice of therapy depends on the specific characteristics of the scar and the patient's preferences.
5. **How do keloid scars differ from hypertrophic scars?**
   Hypertrophic scars remain confined to the wound incision, whereas keloid scars extend beyond the incisional site.
6. **In what scenarios is Z-plasty preferred for scar revision?**
   Z-plasty is favoured when a change in the direction of a scar is necessary, functioning as a transpositional flap. The required change in direction impacts the length of the scar, with every 15 degrees of angle change necessitating a 25% increase in scar length to achieve the desired adjustment.
7. **What are the non-surgical management options for keloids?**

Non-surgical treatments for keloids include intralesional injections of steroids like triamcinolone acetonide (10–40 mg/mL), which can be repeated every 4–6 weeks for up to five doses. Other options include retinoic acid; interferon (IFN) therapy; botulinum toxin; chemotherapy agents such as bleomycin, verapamil, and 5-fluorouracil (5-FU); radiotherapy for resistant cases with a low dose of radiation (15–30 Gy); and UVB therapy.

8. **What surgical options are considered for keloid removal?**
   Surgical approaches to keloid removal can involve intralesional or extralesional excision; laser therapy using devices like diode, KTP, or CO_2 lasers; and cryosurgery.

7.4 Blepharoplasty (Upper and Lower Eyelid Surgery)

Indications for Surgery [3]

- Excess skin or fat in the upper or lower eyelids
- Hooding of the upper eyelid affecting vision
- Aesthetic concerns due to ageing or hereditary factors
- Lower eyelid bags or wrinkles
- Eyelid malposition (e.g. ectropion, entropion)

Risks Involved with the Surgery [3]

- Bleeding
- Infection
- Scarring
- Asymmetry or unsatisfactory cosmetic result:
  - Altered eye shape
  - Eyelid malposition
  - Rounder lid appearance
- Injury to the eye or surrounding structures
- Dry eye or excessive tearing
- Scleral show
- Ectropion
- Corneal abrasions
- Diplopia
- Orbital compartment syndrome

Upper Eyelid Blepharoplasty (see Fig. 7.5)

1. Preoperative planning:
   - Conduct a detailed examination of the patient's eyelid anatomy, focusing on skin quality, fat distribution, and muscle tone.

Fig. 7.5 Upper eyelid blepharoplasty. Illustrated by Vikum Liyanaarachchi

1. Upper eye sagging

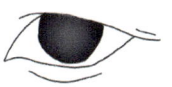

2. Full incision is made along eye crease

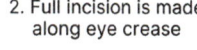
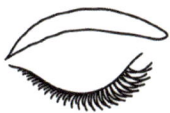

3. Excess tissue is removed

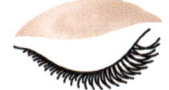

4. Remaining tissue is corrected by lifting

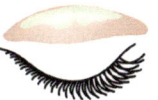

5. Suture along crease

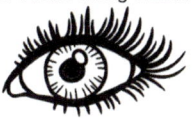

- Discuss the patient's aesthetic and functional goals, assessing any vision impairment due to excess eyelid skin.
- Mark the eyelid with precise measurements, indicating incision lines along the natural crease and delineating the exact amount of skin and potential fat to be removed.

2. Anaesthesia:
   - Administer local anaesthesia, typically a combination of lidocaine and epinephrine, to numb the upper eyelid area. Sedation may be added for patient comfort.
   - In certain cases, general anaesthesia might be used, especially if the patient has specific medical conditions or preferences.
3. Incision:
   - Make a precise incision along the pre-marked crease of the upper eyelid, ensuring minimal visibility of the scar post-surgery.
   - Incise through the skin and orbicularis oculi muscle to expose underlying fat pads and the orbital septum.
4. Skin and Fat Removal:
   - Carefully excise the predetermined amount of excess skin using surgical scissors.
   - Identify and conservatively remove or reposition excess orbital fat, paying attention to avoid hollowing of the eyelid.
5. Closure:
   - Suture the incision meticulously, typically using fine, absorbable sutures to minimize scarring.
   - Apply a small amount of antibiotic ointment to the suture line.
   - Place a light, non-compressive dressing over the eyelids.

Lower Eyelid Blepharoplasty

1. Preoperative planning:
   - Evaluate the lower eyelid's anatomy, noting skin laxity, fat prolapse, and overall eyelid tone.
   - Discuss aesthetic goals, particularly addressing under-eye bags, wrinkles, and dark circles.
   - Mark incision lines carefully, considering the patient's unique eyelid structure.
2. Anaesthesia:
   - Administer local anaesthesia (with or without sedation) or general anaesthesia, based on the patient's health and comfort levels.
3. Incision:
   - Choose the incision technique:
   - Subciliary approach: Make an incision just below the lash line for direct access to excess skin and fat.
   - Transconjunctival approach: Incise inside the lower eyelid, targeting fat without visible scars.
4. Fat Removal or Repositioning:
   - Carefully remove or reposition fat to smooth out bulges and improve contour.
   - Pay attention to maintaining a natural under-eye appearance, avoiding over-removal of fat.
5. Skin removal (if Needed):
   - If using the subciliary approach, precisely remove excess skin, taking care not to over-tighten the eyelid.
6. Closure:
   - For subciliary incisions, use fine sutures for closure, ensuring a well-aligned and discreet scar.
   - In the transconjunctival approach, the incision may be left to heal naturally without sutures.
   - Apply antibiotic ointment and a protective, light dressing to the area.

Important Points to Note During the Surgery

- Preserve the structural integrity of the eyelid to prevent post-operative complications such as eyelid malposition or dry eye.
- Minimize tissue trauma and maintain good haemostasis to reduce post-operative swelling and bruising.
- Tailor the surgical approach and technique to the patient's specific anatomy and goals to achieve the best cosmetic result.

Questions a Consultant Might Ask a Trainee About the Operation

1. **How do you determine the amount of skin to be removed in an upper eyelid blepharoplasty?**

The amount of skin to be removed should be based on the patient's anatomy, goals, and expectations. While the patient is sitting upright, the surgeon should mark the incision lines, ensuring that enough skin is preserved for proper eyelid closure and function.
2. **What are the advantages and disadvantages of the subciliary and transconjunctival approaches for lower eyelid blepharoplasty?**

    The subciliary approach allows for removal of excess skin and fat but may have a higher risk of eyelid malposition or scarring. The transconjunctival approach avoids visible external scarring and has a lower risk of eyelid malposition but does not address excess skin.
3. **How do you manage complications such as dry eye or ectropion after blepharoplasty?**

    Dry eye can be managed with conservative measures, such as lubricating eye drops, ointments, or punctal plugs. Ectropion may require conservative measures such as massage, taping, or temporary eyelid tacking. In some cases, surgical revision may be necessary to address the underlying cause, such as excessive skin removal or scarring.
4. **What factors should be considered when choosing between local anaesthesia with sedation and general anaesthesia for blepharoplasty?**

    Factors to consider include the patient's preference, medical history, extent of the surgery, and the surgeon's experience and preference. Local anaesthesia with sedation may offer quicker recovery and fewer side effects, while general anaesthesia may be more appropriate for patients with anxiety or more extensive procedures.

7.5 Rhytidectomy (Facelift)

Indications for Surgery [4]

- Sagging facial skin and soft tissues due to ageing or weight loss
- Deep facial wrinkles or folds (e.g. nasolabial folds, marionette lines)
- Jowls or loss of jawline definition
- Loose or sagging neck skin

Specific Risks Involved with the Surgery [4]

- Bleeding
- Infection
- Scarring
- Nerve injury (e.g. facial nerve or sensory nerves)
- Asymmetry or unsatisfactory cosmetic result
- Haematoma or seroma
- Skin necrosis or hair loss along the incision
- Anaesthesia complications

Steps of the Surgery

1. Preoperative planning: Assess the patient's anatomy, goals, and expectations. Develop a surgical plan, including the choice of incision and the extent of dissection.
2. Anaesthesia: Administer general anaesthesia or local anaesthesia with sedation, depending on patient preference and medical factors.
3. Incision: Make incisions typically starting at the temple, extending in front of the ear, around the earlobe, and then behind the ear into the hairline (Fig. 7.6).
4. Skin and soft tissue dissection: Elevate the skin and soft tissues in the subcutaneous or sub-SMAS (superficial musculoaponeurotic system) plane, depending on the surgical plan.
5. SMAS manipulation: Tighten the SMAS layer by plication, imbrication, or SMASectomy, as appropriate.
6. Skin redraping and excision: Redrape the skin, removing any excess to achieve a natural and rejuvenated appearance.
7. Closure: Close the incisions with sutures, staples, or tissue adhesives, ensuring good apposition of the wound edges. Apply a light dressing and compression garment.

Important Points to Note During the Surgery

- Preserve the integrity of the facial nerve and sensory nerves to minimize the risk of nerve injury.
- Ensure proper haemostasis to reduce the risk of haematoma or seroma formation.
- Avoid excessive tension on the skin closure to minimize the risk of scarring or skin necrosis.
- Rhytidectomy techniques vary based on the extent of ageing signs and patient needs, including the short flap rhytidectomy (mini lift), subcutaneous rhytidectomy (long flap technique), SMAS technique, deep plane technique, subperiosteal technique, and suture lift (thread lift). Each technique offers different benefits and is chosen based on individual patient characteristics.

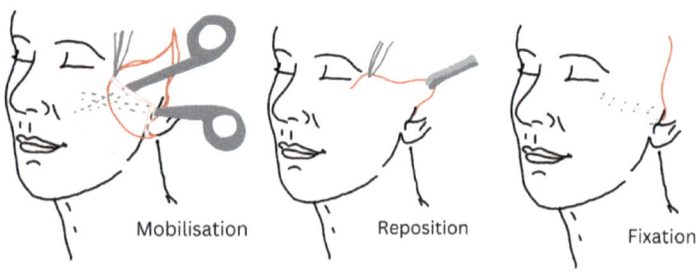

Fig. 7.6 Example of facelift incision and technique. Illustrated by Vikum Liyanaarachchi

Questions a Consultant Might Ask a Trainee About the Operation

1. **How do you choose between a subcutaneous and a sub-SMAS dissection for a facelift?**
   The choice depends on the patient's anatomy, goals, and the surgeon's experience and preference. Subcutaneous dissection is less invasive and may be suitable for patients with mild-to-moderate ageing changes but may not provide as durable or significant a lift as sub-SMAS dissection. Sub-SMAS dissection can provide more substantial and long-lasting results but may have a higher risk of complications, such as nerve injury.
2. **What are the key landmarks for identifying the facial nerve during a facelift?**
   Key landmarks include the tragal pointer (anterior to the ear canal), the posterior belly of the digastric muscle, and the angle of the mandible. The facial nerve typically emerges from the parotid gland at the level of the tragal pointer and divides into its main branches within the parotid gland.
3. **How do you manage a haematoma after a facelift?**
   Haematomas should be promptly recognized and managed to prevent complications, such as infection or skin necrosis. Small haematomas may be managed conservatively with compression and close observation. Larger haematomas may require surgical evacuation and exploration to identify and control any bleeding sources.
4. **How do you minimize the risk of scarring or hair loss along the incision line in a facelift?**
   To minimize scarring, use meticulous dissection techniques, avoid excessive tension on the skin closure, and ensure good apposition of the wound edges. To minimize hair loss, make incisions within the hair-bearing skin and preserve hair follicles during dissection and closure.
5. **How can you achieve a natural-appearing result in a facelift?**
   Achieving a natural result requires careful preoperative planning, individualized surgical techniques, and attention to detail. Preserve the patient's unique facial features, and avoid excessive tightening or overcorrection. Focus on addressing the underlying facial soft tissues (e.g. SMAS layer) rather than just tightening the skin, to create a more youthful and balanced appearance.
6. **Which patients do you avoid performing this on?**
   Smoker who has lost weight, uncontrolled BP/DM, active skin conditions, and one who has unreasonable expectations

7.6 Brow Lift (Endoscopic, Direct, Mid-Forehead)

Indications for Surgery

- Forehead wrinkles or deep furrows
- Sagging or low-positioned eyebrows
- Hooding of the upper eyelids due to brow ptosis
- Aesthetic concerns related to the appearance of the forehead and eyebrows

Specific Risks Involved with the Surgery

- Bleeding
- Infection
- Scarring
- Nerve injury (e.g. frontal branch of the facial nerve or sensory nerves)
- Asymmetry or unsatisfactory cosmetic result
- Hair loss or hairline changes
- Anaesthesia complications

Steps of the Surgery

Endoscopic Brow Lift
1. Preoperative planning: Assess the patient's anatomy, goals, and expectations. Mark the incision sites.
2. Anaesthesia: Administer general anaesthesia or local anaesthesia with sedation, depending on patient preference and medical factors.
3. Incision: Make several small incisions within the hair-bearing scalp, avoiding visible scarring.
4. Dissection and elevation: Use an endoscope and specialized instruments to dissect the forehead tissues and elevate the brow.
5. Fixation: Secure the elevated brow position with sutures, screws, or other fixation devices.
6. Closure: Close the incisions with sutures, staples, or tissue adhesives. Apply a light dressing.

Direct Brow Lift
1. Preoperative planning: As with the endoscopic approach, assess the patient's anatomy, goals, and expectations. Mark the incision sites.
2. Anaesthesia: Administer local anaesthesia with or without sedation, or general anaesthesia.
3. Incision: Make an incision along the upper edge of the eyebrow or within a forehead crease.
4. Dissection and elevation: Dissect the forehead tissues and elevate the brow.
5. Fixation: Suture the elevated brow position to the underlying periosteum.
6. Closure: Close the incision with sutures, ensuring good apposition of the wound edges. Apply a light dressing.

Mid-Forehead Brow Lift
1. Preoperative planning: As with the other approaches, assess the patient's anatomy, goals, and expectations. Mark the incision sites.

2. Anaesthesia: Administer local anaesthesia with or without sedation or general anaesthesia.
3. Incision: Make an incision within a deep forehead crease or wrinkle.
4. Dissection and elevation: Dissect the forehead tissues, and elevate the brow.
5. Fixation: Suture the elevated brow position to the underlying periosteum.
6. Closure: Close the incision with sutures, ensuring good apposition of the wound edges. Apply a light dressing.

Important Points to Note During the Surgery

- Preserve the integrity of the facial nerve branches and sensory nerves to minimize the risk of nerve injury.
- Choose the appropriate surgical approach based on the patient's anatomy, goals, and surgeon's experience.
- Ensure proper haemostasis to reduce the risk of haematoma or seroma formation.
- Brow lift techniques range from minimally invasive to more comprehensive procedures, including Botox (chemical brow lift), browpexy, direct brow lift, endoscopic brow lift, mid-forehead lift, trichophytic forehead lift, and coronal forehead lift. The choice of technique is dependent on the desired outcome and anatomical considerations.

Questions a Consultant Might Ask a Trainee About the Operation

1. **How do you determine the ideal brow position during a brow lift?**
   The ideal brow position depends on the patient's anatomy, goals, and expectations. In general, the brow should be positioned above the supraorbital rim, with the lateral brow higher than the medial brow. The surgeon should also consider the patient's desired brow shape and arch.
2. **What are the advantages and disadvantages of the endoscopic, direct, and mid-forehead brow lift approaches?**
   The endoscopic approach is less invasive, with smaller incisions and reduced scarring, but may not provide as substantial a lift as the other approaches. The direct and mid-forehead approaches provide more significant and durable results but have more visible scarring. The direct approach is well suited for patients with heavy brows or lateral brow ptosis, while the mid-forehead approach is suitable for patients with high hairlines or deep forehead wrinkles.
3. **How do you manage complications such as nerve injury or unsatisfactory cosmetic results after a brow lift?**
   For nerve injuries, conservative management with observation and time may allow for nerve recovery. In some cases, additional surgery may be required for nerve repair or to address the cause of the injury. Unsatisfactory cosmetic results may be addressed through revision surgery, taking into account the specific concerns and patient goals.

4. **How do you minimize hair loss or hairline changes after a brow lift?**
   To minimize hair loss or hairline changes, make incisions within the hair-bearing skin and preserve hair follicles during dissection and closure. Choose the appropriate surgical approach based on the patient's hairline, anatomy, and goals.
5. **How do you decide between general anaesthesia and local anaesthesia with sedation for a brow lift?**
   Factors to consider include the patient's preference, medical history, extent of the surgery, and the surgeon's experience and preference. Local anaesthesia with sedation may offer quicker recovery and fewer side effects, while general anaesthesia may be more appropriate for patients with anxiety or more extensive procedures.

7.7 Genioplasty (Chin Augmentation/Reduction)

Indications for Surgery

- Retrognathia or micrognathia (small or receding chin)
- Prognathism (prominent or protruding chin)
- Asymmetrical chin
- Aesthetic concerns related to the size, shape, or position of the chin

Specific Risks Involved with the Surgery

- Bleeding
- Infection
- Scarring
- Nerve injury (e.g. mental nerve)
- Bone resorption or malunion
- Asymmetry or unsatisfactory cosmetic result
- Anaesthesia complications

Steps of the Surgery

1. Preoperative planning:
2. Detailed assessment:
   - Conduct a comprehensive evaluation of the patient's facial anatomy, focusing on the chin's size, projection, and symmetry relative to other facial features.
   - Utilize imaging studies, like cephalometric analysis or 3D imaging, to assess the bony anatomy and plan the osteotomy precisely.

Fig. 7.7 Intraoral incision. Illustrated by Vikum Liyanaarachchi

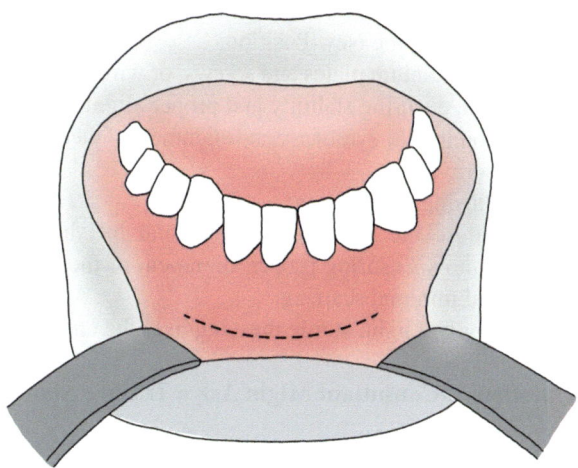

- Discuss the patient's aesthetic goals, such as enhancing chin projection or reducing chin prominence, and manage expectations realistically.
3. Marking the Incision Site:
    - If opting for an intraoral approach, mark the incision line along the gingivolabial sulcus (the crease where the lower lip and gums meet). See Fig. 7.7.
    - For an external approach, mark a discreet incision site under the chin.
4. Anaesthesia:
    - Depending on the complexity of the procedure and patient preference, choose between general anaesthesia (for more extensive manipulation or patient comfort) and local anaesthesia with sedation.
5. Incision:
    - Perform an intraoral incision along the marked gingivolabial sulcus to access the chin bone without visible scarring.
    - Alternatively, make a submental incision (under the chin) for direct access, especially in cases requiring significant manipulation or when an extraoral approach is preferred.
6. Dissection:
    Elevating soft tissues:
    - Carefully dissect the soft tissues, including muscles and connective tissues, to expose the chin bone (mandible) while minimizing damage to surrounding structures.
7. Osteotomy:
8. Performing the Bone Cut:
    - Execute a precise horizontal osteotomy (bone cut) on the mandible according to the preoperative plan.
    - Depending on the desired outcome, either slide the chin bone segment forward (for augmentation) or backward or reduce its height (for reduction).

9. Fixation:
   Securing the New Position:
   - Use titanium plates and screws, or wires, to fix the chin bone in its new position, ensuring stability and proper alignment with the rest of the jaw.
   - Confirm the symmetry and alignment of the chin relative to other facial features.
10. Closure:
    Closing the incision:
    - Suture the intraoral or submental incision meticulously with absorbable sutures, ensuring proper alignment of the wound edges for optimal healing and minimal scarring.
    - Apply a light, sterile dressing over the chin area.

Questions a Consultant Might Ask a Trainee About the Operation

1. **What are the key anatomical landmarks to consider during genioplasty?**
   Key landmarks include the mental foramen, the mental nerve, the inferior border of the mandible, and the midline of the chin. Proper identification and preservation of these structures are crucial for achieving a successful outcome and minimizing the risk of complications.
2. **How do you determine the ideal position of the chin during genioplasty?**
   The ideal position of the chin depends on the patient's anatomy, goals, and expectations. Preoperative imaging and simulations can help guide the planning process. The chin should be positioned in a way that creates a harmonious facial profile and balances the patient's other facial features.
3. **How do you manage complications such as nerve injury, bone resorption, or unsatisfactory cosmetic results after genioplasty?**
   For nerve injuries, conservative management with observation and time may allow for nerve recovery. In some cases, additional surgery may be required for nerve repair or to address the cause of the injury. Bone resorption may be managed with bone grafting or revision surgery. Unsatisfactory cosmetic results may be addressed through revision surgery, considering the specific concerns and patient goals.
4. **How do you minimize the risk of infection or scarring during genioplasty?**
   To minimize the risk of infection, maintain strict aseptic technique, use appropriate perioperative antibiotics, and ensure proper wound care postoperatively. To minimize scarring, choose the appropriate incision location (intraoral or submental) based on the patient's anatomy and goals, and use meticulous dissection and closure techniques.
5. **When should a sliding genioplasty be considered over a chin implant for chin augmentation?**
   A sliding genioplasty may be more appropriate for patients with significant chin deformities, vertical height discrepancies, or asymmetry that cannot be adequately addressed with a chin implant. It can also be used in cases where precise control over the chin position is required or when the patient prefers an autologous procedure.

7.8 Facial Implants (Cheek, Jaw, Temporal)

Indications for Surgery

- Flat or underdeveloped cheekbones
- Weak or underdeveloped jawline
- Aesthetic concerns related to the size, shape, or position of facial structures
- Facial asymmetry or contour irregularities

Specific Risks Involved with the Surgery

- Bleeding
- Infection
- Scarring
- Nerve injury (e.g. facial or sensory nerves)
- Implant malposition, extrusion, or migration
- Asymmetry or unsatisfactory cosmetic result
- Anaesthesia complications

Steps of the Surgery

1. Preoperative planning: Assess the patient's anatomy, goals, and expectations. Select the appropriate implant size and shape.
2. Anaesthesia: Administer general anaesthesia or local anaesthesia with sedation, depending on patient preference and medical factors.
3. Incision: Make incisions in inconspicuous locations, such as inside the mouth, within the hairline, or along natural skin creases.
4. Dissection: Create a pocket between the bone and soft tissue to accommodate the implant.
5. Implant placement: Insert the implant into the pocket and ensure proper positioning. See Fig. 7.8 for examples.
6. Fixation (if needed): Secure the implant in place with sutures or screws.
7. Closure: Close the incision with sutures, ensuring good apposition of the wound edges. Apply a light dressing.

Important Points to Note During the Surgery

- Preserve the integrity of facial nerves and blood vessels to minimize the risk of nerve injury or bleeding.
- Ensure proper implant sizing and positioning to achieve a natural and aesthetically pleasing result.
- Use meticulous dissection and closure techniques to minimize scarring and reduce the risk of infection or implant extrusion.

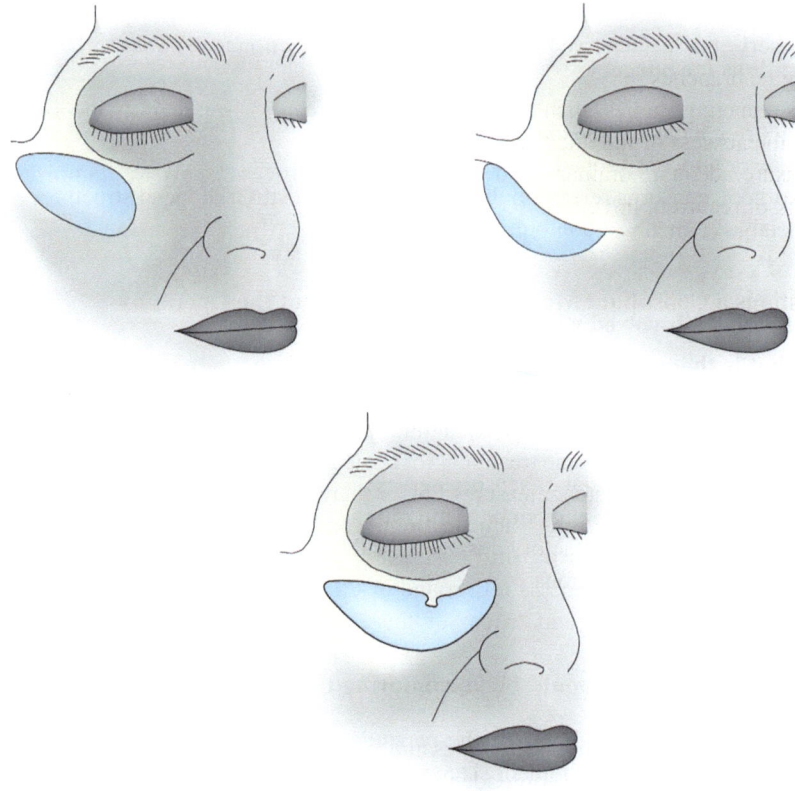

Fig. 7.8 Examples of cheek implants. Illustrated by Vikum Liyanaarachchi

Questions a Consultant Might Ask a Trainee About the Operation

1. **What are the different types of implant material used:**
   When considering facial implants, material choices include metals like gold and titanium; polymers such as silicone; biodegradable options like PDS; injectable implants like Sculptra; and biologic implants, including fat, cartilage, bone, nerve, and allograft. The material selection depends on the specific requirements of the augmentation and patient preferences.
2. **What are the advantages and disadvantages of using autologous grafts (e.g., fat, bone) compared to synthetic implants for facial augmentation?**
   Autologous grafts have the advantages of being biocompatible and less likely to cause an immune response and can integrate well with the surrounding tissues. However, they may be subject to resorption or unpredictable volume changes over time. Synthetic implants provide a more predictable and stable result but carry a risk of infection, extrusion, or malposition.

3. **How do you minimize the risk of nerve injury during facial implant surgery?**
   To minimize nerve injury, identify and preserve facial nerves during dissection, use blunt dissection techniques, and ensure that the implant does not apply excessive pressure on the nerves.
4. **How do you decide between general anaesthesia and local anaesthesia with sedation for facial implant surgery?**
   Factors to consider include the patient's preference, medical history, extent of the surgery, and the surgeon's experience and preference. Local anaesthesia with sedation may offer quicker recovery and fewer side effects, while general anaesthesia may be more appropriate for patients with anxiety or more extensive procedures.

7.9 Lip Augmentation/Reduction

Indications for Surgery

- Thin or underdeveloped lips
- Overly large or protruding lips
- Asymmetrical lips
- Aesthetic concerns related to the size, shape, or position of the lips

Specific Risks Involved with the Surgery

- Bleeding
- Infection
- Scarring
- Nerve injury (e.g. labial nerves)
- Asymmetry or unsatisfactory cosmetic result
- Anaesthesia complications

Steps of the Surgery

1. Preoperative planning: Assess the patient's anatomy, goals, and expectations. Mark the incision site and desired lip contour.
2. Anaesthesia: Administer local anaesthesia with or without sedation, depending on patient preference and medical factors.
3. Incision: Make incisions along the vermilion border or inside the lip, depending on the specific technique being used.
4. Tissue manipulation: For augmentation, inject dermal fillers and autologous fat or place lip implants. For reduction, excise excess tissue and reshape the lip as needed. See Fig. 7.9.
5. Closure: Close the incision with sutures, ensuring good apposition of the wound edges. Apply a light dressing.

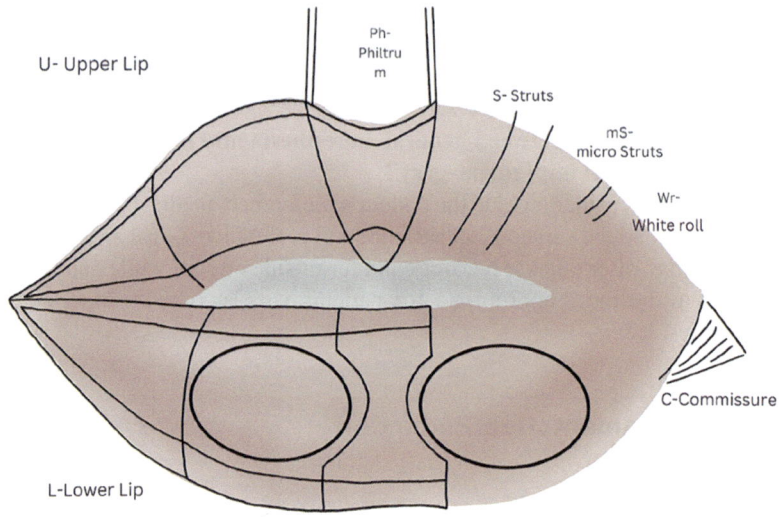

Fig. 7.9 Lip anatomy and zones. Illustrated by Vikum Liyanaarachchi

Important Points to Note for Surgery

- Lip augmentation and reduction techniques are varied to suit patient needs and include the use of autologous materials like fat and SMAS; fillers such as HA; implants like Alloderm and silicone; and surgical methods including V-Y advancement, double Y-V mucosal plasty, and vermillion advancement excision. Reduction techniques include vermillion reduction and bikini lip reduction.

Questions a Consultant Might Ask a Trainee About the Operation

1. **What are the key principles for achieving natural-looking results with lip fillers?**
   Aim for natural-looking lip enhancements by following the golden ratio, aiming for a 1:1.6 proportion between the upper and lower lip for balance. Key guidelines include ensuring symmetry, enhancing the vermilion border and Cupid's bow for definition, maintaining natural texture and movement, and considering age-related changes. Overfilling can lead to stiffness and an unnatural appearance.
2. **What factors should be considered when deciding between autologous fat grafting, dermal fillers, or lip implants for lip augmentation?**
   Factors to consider include the patient's preference, medical history, desired lip size and shape, and the surgeon's experience and preference. Autologous fat grafting is biocompatible and may provide a more natural appearance but can have unpredictable results. Dermal fillers offer a minimally invasive option with

immediate results but may require regular maintenance. Lip implants provide a more permanent solution but carry a risk of infection, extrusion, or malposition.
3. **When should a patient consider lip reduction surgery?**
   A patient may consider lip reduction surgery if they have overly large or protruding lips that cause functional issues (e.g. difficulty eating or speaking) or aesthetic concerns. The decision to undergo lip reduction surgery should be based on the patient's goals, expectations, and a thorough discussion with the surgeon about the potential risks and benefits.

References

1. Naumann A. Otoplasty–techniques, characteristics and risks. GMS Curr Top Otorhinolaryngol Head Neck Surg. 2007;6:Doc04.
2. Bailey JS, Goldwasser MS. Surgical management of facial skin cancer. Oral Maxillofac Surg Clin North Am. 2005;17(2):205–33.
3. Naik MN, Honavar SG, Das S, Desai S, Dhepe N. Blepharoplasty: an overview. J Cutan Aesthet Surg. 2009;2(1):6–11.
4. Barrett DM, Casanueva FJ, Wang TD. Evolution of the rhytidectomy. World J Otorhinolaryngol Head Neck Surg. 2016;2(1):38–44.

GPSR Compliance

The European Union's (EU) General Product Safety Regulation (GPSR) is a set of rules that requires consumer products to be safe and our obligations to ensure this.

If you have any concerns about our products, you can contact us on ProductSafety@springernature.com

In case Publisher is established outside the EU, the EU authorized representative is:

Springer Nature Customer Service Center GmbH
Europaplatz 3
69115 Heidelberg, Germany

Batch number: 09151316

Printed by Printforce, the Netherlands